New
Exercises
for Runners

By the Editors of *Runner's World*

World Publications, Inc.
Mountain View, CA 94042

Recommended Reading:
Runner's World Magazine, $13.00/year
Write for a free catalog of publications
and supplies for runners and other athletes.

Library of Congress 78-460
ISBN 0-89307-151-2

Contents

Foreword

Like many runners with roots in the 1950s and '60s, I once thought exercises were a waste of time. The calisthenics of football and Army basic training were used more to discipline the mind than train the body, and we runners already had plenty of self-discipline. Hurdlers and sprinters may have needed these contortions, but distance runners' time was better spent running.

I thought I put extra exercises behind me when I stopped playing football at 18, starting up again only for a few unpleasant months in the Army at 22. For almost 10 years after that, I didn't do a pushup, situp or toetouch. It was too much like work, and it would have taken away from the fun of running.

Meanwhile, injuries began to nag at me—little ones at first, the kind that don't stop you but nibble away at the joy of moving freely. I ignored these little hurts, and they grew into big ones—the kind that cause you to miss a day here and there, then several days, then whole weeks. Eventually, I ran myself into foot surgery—and still hadn't figured out why.

George Sheehan told me why. Dr. Sheehan, the medical columnist and philosopher-in-residence of *Runner's World,* casually tosses off lines that are the envy of anyone who writes. His wisdom comes in the form of short, simple, flat statements, which are easy to read and hard to forget.

The Sheehan "proverb" that fits the subject of runners' exercises concerns strength and flexibility. He said, "Joe, when you run, three things happen and two of them are bad."

He means physical things. The good one is that you become a faster and more enduring runner; you adapt to the kind of exercise you do. But if you don't do any exercise except run, the bad things happen and may—in extreme cases—stop you from running as they progress. The first of these is tightness of the backside, all the way from the heels to the lower back, unless you're doing corrective exercises. If you're a longtime long-distance runner, you probably can't bend from the waist with your knees straight and touch your fingertips to the ground.

The second bad effect is loss of muscle strength in the upper body and development of strength imbalances in the legs. Runners' arms, shoulders, chest and abdominal muscles are pretty much just along for the ride; if they're neglected, they shrink. The front-of-leg muscles from the hip on down get worked, but not as hard as the ones in back; this accounts for the imbalances.

At best, then, runners aren't as fit as they like to believe if they lack flexibility and strength. At worst, they're wide open to all kinds of injuries.

I found the injuries, as hundreds of other runners have, when I specialized too much on running. (This is particularly true for those of us who do little or no speed training; faster running returns some of the strength and flexibility that long, slower distance takes away.) I now know that exercises are a good investment, giving hours of smooth running for a few minutes of supplemental work. I invest in it every day and now tell other runners to do the same.

But even if you never get hurt, there is another and more positive reason to exercise: *performance.* You can run faster with the same or less effort if you're loose and strong. The stride is freer and has more power behind it—factors that aren't necessarily enhanced by running alone.

Try this: First, bend over and touch the ground (even if only with the fingertips). Then, do 10 *honest* pushups and bent-leg situps. If you can't pass these minimum tests of flexibility and strength, or if leg injuries are eroding the fun of your running, you need this book.

Joe Henderson

I
Testing Yourself

1

Running's Bad Results

George Sheehan, M.D.

When an athlete goes into training, three things can happen to his muscles. Two of them are bad: shortening of the strengthened muscles with loss of flexibility; weakness of the opposing, relatively unused muscles.

"The irony is that the athlete is less fit in regard to flexibility standards than the typical man in the street," writes *Fitness for Living* editor Robert Bahr. "That's because strengthening and endurance exercises act to shorten muscles and reduce flexibility." It is Bahr's belief also that most muscle tears, pulls and strains occur because of this lack of flexibility.

The best answer to this lack of flexibility is yoga. For one thing, in yoga the stretching is gentle, smooth, nonpainful and achieved over a period of time. "Stretching by bobbing or bouncing," writes physiologist Dr. Herbert de Vries, "invokes the stretch reflex which actually opposes the desired stretching."

Yoga or not, the stretching athlete is only halfway home. He has to start strengthening exercises of the weakened antagonist muscles. This will prevent the imbalance in muscle strength that many observers feel is the other major cause of pulls, tears and strains.

"A number of studies have shown," says physiotherapist Joseph Zohar, "that when one muscle group is excessively stronger than the opposing muscle group, the odds of injury in the weaker muscle are greatly increased." The evidence is that an excessively high ratio of strength between the

---

Dr. **Sheehan,** heart specialist, runner, and writer, is the medical editor of *Runner's World* magazine. At age 59, he still races regularly—including running the Boston Marathon each year. He is author of *Dr. Sheehan On Running* (Mountain View, Calif.: World Publications, 1975).

quadriceps (the front thigh muscles) and the hamstrings (the rear thigh muscles increases the chance of a hamstring pull.

The principle is easy, the application difficult. Each sport strengthens and therefore shortens a different set of muscles. The flexibility problems of a sprinter, for instance, differ from those of the distance runner, as do his muscle imbalances. The distance runner has stronger, shorter hamstrings and therefore tends to pull his weaker quadriceps. The sprinter who uses his quads to explode out of the blocks has weaker hamstrings, and the back of his thigh is where he grabs when he gets that tearing sensation midway in the 100-yard dash.

The main interest of the people in sports medicine is not to predict these events (which some researchers have done by testing athletes) but to prevent them. This biomechanical approach to muscle balance provides just such a program. It is part yoga, part muscle balancing. Zohar calls it preventive conditioning. What it means is that no weakness, no tightness, no muscle imbalance will go uncorrected.

When an athlete trains that way, when he applies engineering and architectural principles to his body, he doesn't have to worry about the two bad things that usually happen. And he may even get some unexpected dividends.

"The balanced conditioning of individual muscle groups," states Zohar, "not only protects the body against injury but also improves its performance to unprecedented levels."

But before you can start stretching and strengthening, you need to find out where you are tight or out of balance, what you can do to correct the irregularities and what bonus or side-effects you can expect.

2

See Where You Stand

Can you touch your toes?

Put this book aside, stand up, knees straight, feet together, and bend forward slowly and carefully. Reach down with your fingertips until the muscles tighten in the backs of your legs.

If you're a runner, have been for some time but have not been doing flexibility work for that time, you're probably hung up somewhere along the shinbone between the knee and the ankle. Don't feel bad. You aren't alone. Running does this to people, and the simple toe- or floor-touch is the most telling evidence that they haven't taken corrective measures against tightening.

Most runners are overly tight in the legs. Dr. Steven Subotnick, a podiatrist with a large athlete clientele, says the trait is almost universal in his runner-patients. He says nine in 10 of them can't pass minimum tests of flexibility. Dr. Subotnick thinks this is one of the main reasons runners come to see him in such numbers.

"The runner," Subotnick says, "must be aware of the fact that strengthening and endurance exercises reduce their flexibility. Long- and middle-distance running result in overdeveloping of the muscles at the back of the lower leg and thigh, in particular the gastrocnemius and soleus in the lower leg, and the hamstring in the thigh."

The doctor says the need for exercises to counteract this tightening "cannot be overstressed." Running muscles are chronically pounded and tensed. They must be fully stretched and relaxed, too, and this doesn't happen while running.

Robert Bahr of *Fitness for Living* magazine writes, "When muscles are forced to contract regularly, the facial sheath that covers the muscles and the sarcolemma of the muscle fiber tend to shorten.... When there is no effort to maintain

6

flexibility, tendons and ligaments also shorten with the passing of time. Occasionally, calcium deposits may build up in the joints, further restricting movement."

Chronically tense, chronically short muscles don't work as they should. They come to restrict the running motion, and predispose the runner to injury.

Dr. Hans Kraus, a pioneer in fitness testing, says that "a muscle must relax. Relaxing is part of its function. If a muscle fails to relax, it stays tight. It loses its stretch, its suppleness, its give. Over a period of time, it becomes permanently shortened. When this happens, a muscle loses most of its ability to relax."

At that point, an individual—regardless of the specific conditioning he thinks he has—is "unfit" by Dr. Kraus's standards. An athlete who can run a mile under five minutes or a marathon under three hours may not even by able to bend over and touch his toes. That is the cost of overspecialized development. The bill is often paid in pain.

Robert Bahr points out, "The irony is that, all other things being equal, [this type of athlete] actually becomes less fit in regard to flexibility than the typical man in the street."

Dr. Kraus adds, "We would feel that these individuals, even though they are extremely 'fit' for their particular endeavors, are not desirably fit from the overall health point of view—and (are) more exposed to muscle strains than their more flexible counterparts."

The same is true when certain running muscles grow powerful with use, while opposing ones required for a healthy balance are allowed to go flabby from neglect. We'll get into particular leg muscle problems in Part III. But here let's talk about the stomach—more precisely, the abdominal muscles. These are a little-recognized source of trouble.

Put the book aside again. Lie down and do a sit-up. Can you do an honest one without straining? Many runners can't according to Dr. George Sheehan, because their abdominals are weak in comparison to the back muscles. When this happens, the spine can be tugged out of alignment, leading to one of the most persistent and dreaded of runner complaints: sciatica. Sharp pains originate in the small of the back and shoot down the legs.

The floor-touch and the sit-up are two of the six Kraus-Weber tests. Drs. Hans Kraus and Sonja Weber devised the tests to measure strength and flexibility. (See the accompanying photos.)

Kraus says the simple exercises "are designed to test the key muscle groups in your body, no matter what your age, height, or weight. These tests are self-correlating. They do not judge you by some outside, arbitrary standard. They do not ask you to be as strong as a coal miner or as lithe as an acrobat. Instead, these tests simply reveal whether or not you have sufficient muscular strength to move your own body weight and the muscular fexibility to match your own size."

If passing these six is a minimum standard for everyday fitness, a runner should have to race through them with ease. Can you? Try all six, exactly as outlined.

"If you passed all six" Kraus says, "you have sufficient strength and flexibility for your weight and height. But if you failed even one of the six you are underexercised or over-tensed, and you need help. In fact, if you had difficulty passing any one of the six tests you should consider yourself below par. This may seem severe or unfair. But you would not be considered healthy if you had perfect vision and hearing, a good pulse rate, but an abnormal red-cell blood count."

Runners apparently are most likely to fail floor-touching and sit-ups. The general public shows the same weaknesses. Kraus notes, "The floor-touch test is failed by a high percentage of patients, and more frequently by men than by women...The weakness of the abdominal muscles is most frequently found in women, especially after pregnancy."

All but the severest cases of weakness and inflexibility are completely reversible through corrective exercises. According to Dr. Kraus, "Your muscles can be trained, if you take the trouble to train them properly. They can become strong and relaxed through purposeful exercise, or they can become shortened and tense from lack of exercise and over-irritation.

3
The Six Tests

"Like mischievous children, muscles are more inclined to stick to bad habits than persist in good ones. How they behave is up to you. Overtensing and shortening of your muscles are very bad habits, and once acquired they may be hard to break."

Breaking old and wrong habits requires doing the right kinds of exercises and doing them regularly. It isn't as simple as doing floor-touches and sit-ups. For one thing, they can be dangerous when done improperly. (They put strain on the lower back in violent, repeated movement. For another, they aren't enough.) Reconditioning requires a well-rounded set of special exercises.

We've been quoting from Dr. Kraus' book, *The Cause, Prevention and Treatment of Backache, Stress and Tension.* Despite its unweildy title, it has good advice for runners. It describes how to devise personal programs, based on individual needs.

Kraus says, "The majority of people do not know what their needs are, yet they buy exercise books and go at the exercises with a vengeance. In doing this, they often injure themselves...I would no more think of telling everyone to do the same set of exercises than your family doctor would tell all his patients—no matter whether they had a broken leg, sinus trouble, or heart disease—to take the same medicine."

With a Kraus-Weber screening, runners can find where or if they need treatment. This is sound preventive medicine.

Test One
Hip-Flexor Strength

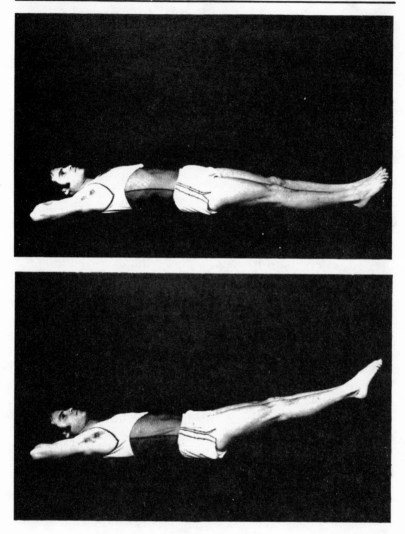

A. Lie on your back, hands clasped behind neck, legs straight and together.

B. Raise straight legs until heels are 10 inches off floor. Hold 10 seconds to pass.

Test Two
Hip-Flexors, Abdominals

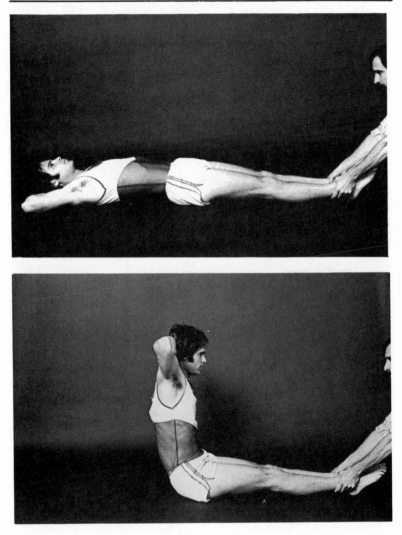

A. Lie on your back, hands clasped behind neck, ankles anchored and legs straight.

B. Sit up to 90-degree angle to pass.

Test Three
Abdominal Strength

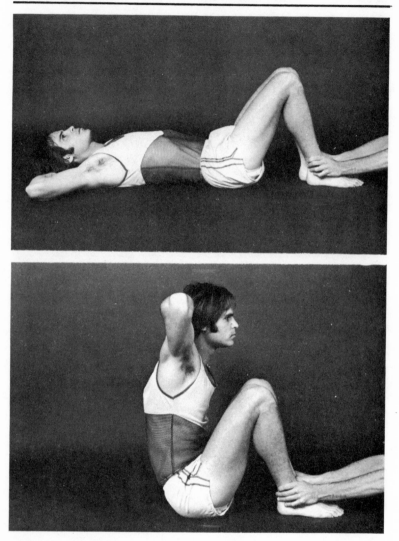

A. Lie on your back, hands clasped behind neck, ankles anchored, knees at about a 90-degree angle.

B. Sit up straight to pass.

Test Four
Upper-Back Strength

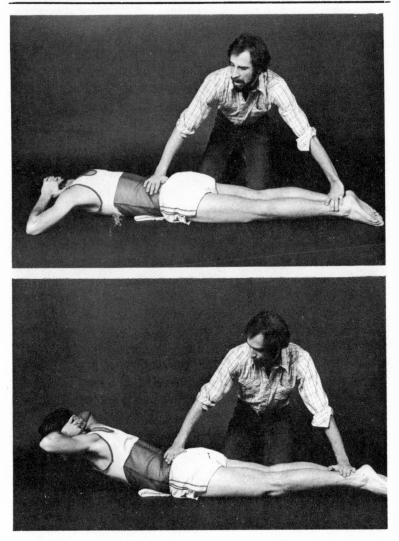

A. Lie on stomach, hands clasped behind neck, pillow under abdomen, ankles and small of back anchored.

B. Lift trunk. Hold for 10 seconds to pass.

Test Five
Lower-Back Strength

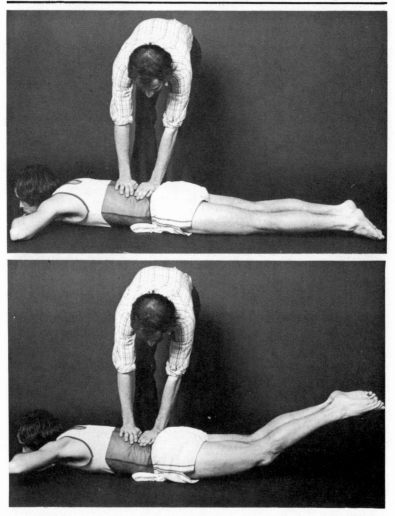

A. Lie on stomach, arms folded under head, pillow under the abdomen, and back anchored.

B. Lift your legs (together). Hold 10 seconds to pass.

Test Six
Leg, Back Flexibility

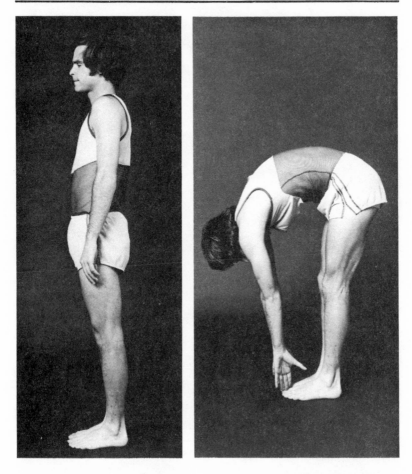

A. Stand up straight, feet together.

B. Bend slowly from waist, knees straight. Touch floor with fingertips to pass.

II
Stretching Exercises

4
Two-Way Stretching

If you think we're about to go into the dreary "hup-two-three-four" routine of high school gym class and army basic training calisthenics, relax. There will be none of that here, for a couple of good reasons.

First, runners instinctively recoil when they hear anyone "hup-two-three-fouring" them. They get enough of this cadence-calling when they're on the streets running, without carrying it over into supplemental stretching exercises. At best, calisthenics that call for a cadence are mechanical, regimented, repetitious movements done more from a feeling of duty than with any real interest or enjoyment.

But more importantly, authorities now are questioning the value of these conventional exercises as a path to flexibility. Robert Bahr, editor of *Fitness for Living,* writes, "The need for flexibility has long been recognized by fitness experts. In both our high schools and the armed services, token recognition of the need for flexibility is given in terms of the calisthenics program. But recent evidence indicates that calisthenics are not advisable for this purpose."

Bahr relies heavily on the evidence of Herbert de Vries, a physiologist at the University of Southern California and author of *Physiology of Exercise for Physical Education and Athletics.*

Dr. de Vries separates stretching exercises into two categories: "ballistic" and "static." Ballistic exercises are the standard vigorous calisthenics. They feature quick, repeated movements. Static exercises involve slow and rhythmic stretching, stopping, and holding a position at the point of first discomfort.

In his Southern California laboratory, de Vries has tried to determine which of the stretching methods is superior. Earlier tests told him "that both slow and fast stretching are effective, and that there is no significant difference between them." He confirmed this in tests of his own, using equivalent ballistic and static exercises.

"It was found," he explains in his book, "that both methods result in significant gains in static flexibility (in seven 30-minute training periods). . . There was no significant difference between methods."

When done properly, the effects of the two appear to be equal. Yet de Vries strongly recommends static stretching. His case is based on "three distinct advantages":

• There is less danger of going beyond the safe limits of stretching because the exerciser moves into position slowly and stops before hurting himself. With ballistic exercises, he may realize too late that he has bounced past his limit.

• Energy costs are lower with static stretching, so the exercises don't tire athletes for other activities.

• Ballistic exercises may cause muscle soreness. Static stretching tends to relieve such soreness.

In short, de Vries prefers static exercises because the effort and the risk are lower. The runner's natural reaction to tiring extra exercise is to avoid it, thereby getting no stretching at all. The natural reaction when doing bouncing-type calisthenics is to bounce too vigorously, thereby defeating the purpose of the exercise.

De Vries says that when a muscle is jerked into extension, it responds by jerking back and shortening itself again. If this jerking back and forth is too violent, the result is soreness.

According to de Vries, "Activities most likely to result in soreness are: (1) vigorous muscle contractions with a muscle in a shortened condition..., (2) muscle contractions that involve jerky movements..., (3) muscle contractions that involve repetitions of the same movement over a long period of time..., and (4) bouncing-type stretching movements."

He seems to have defined running and the standard calisthenics runners use, calisthenics that may be contributing to inflexibility and soreness rather than counteracting them as intended.

The authors of *Foundations of Conditioning* agree with Dr. de Vries. They offer evidence that violent stretching before athletic events "is a predisposing cause of subsequent muscle injury."

They continue, "Empirical observations of athletes tend to indicate that uncontrolled stretching of a ballistic nature may indeed increase the incidence of pulled or torn muscle tissue rather than decrease their incidence, which is one of the original intents of the use of flexibility exercises in warm-up prior to performance."

When Herbert de Vries was working out his static stretching plan, he took an important clue from swimmers, who are particularly prone to calf cramping.

"Competitive swimmers and swimming coaches know," de Vries says, "that swimmer's cramp (gastrocnemius) is promptly relieved by gently forcing the cramped muscle into the longest possible state and holding it there for a moment.

"It was hypothesized that the simple stretching technique that relieves a swimmer's cramp in the calf muscle should also be effective in providing prevention and relief for any muscle that can be put on stretch."

The hope in stretching is to prevent soreness through adequate flexibility. But any runner knows that some carry-over pain is inevitable in his sport. Methods that can keep pain moderate and flush it out quickly are good enough. And Dr. de Vries has such a method.

He tells athletes to determine which muscle or muscles are involved, find the muscular attachments of the involved muscle or muscles and then "devise a simple position in which the attachments are held as far apart as possible with the lease possible effort...Hold this position for two two-minute periods, with a one-minute rest period intervening. If the pain is severe, this should be repeated two or three times daily. This procedure has been effective even in chronic muscular problems."

DeVries says, "Many yoga exercises have been found useful since they use the same principles." The truth is more likely the reverse. His exercises are effective because they are based on hatha yoga, which is as old as history itself.

5
Six Steps Toward Painless Running
George Sheehan, M.D.

If you want to run a marathon, you must train the Magic Six (miles a day). If you are looking for that natural high distance runners talk about, you must do the same. And if you would prefer to die of something other than a heart attack the daily six miles is the physiological magic.

But know this: Disaster will pursue you to the very gates of this heaven unless you do another Magic Six. These are the Magic Six exercises designed to counteract the bad effects of this daily training—the muscle imbalance that contributes to the overuse syndromes of the foot, leg, knee and low back. Without this Magic Six, you will soon become an ex-runner, no longer able to accept 5000 footstrikes an hour on a hard, flat surface with a foot constructed for sand or dirt.

Training overdevelops the prime movers—those muscles along the back of the leg and thigh and low back become short and inflexible. The antagonists—the muscles on the front of the leg and thigh and abdomen—become relatively weak. The Magic Six are necessary to correct this strength/flexibility imbalance: three to stretch and three to strengthen.

It takes a little over six minutes to do the Magic Six. Done before and after running, this means just 12 minutes a day to keep you in muscle balance.

21

One • Wall Pushup

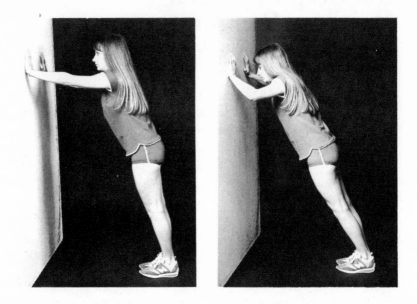

1. The first stretching exercise is the *wall pushup* for the calf muscles. Stand flat-footed about three feet from the wall. Lean in until it hurts, keeping the knees locked, the legs straight and the feet flat. Count "one elephant, two elephants," etc. Hold for 10 elephants. Relax. Repeat for one minute.

Two • Hamstring Stretch

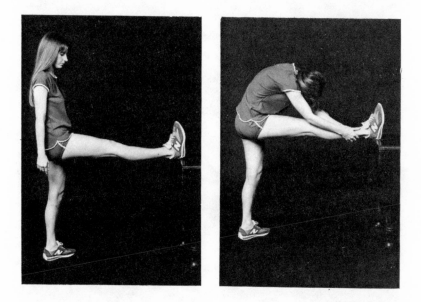

2. The second is the *hamstring stretch*. Put your straight leg with knee locked on a footstool, later a chair, finally a table as you improve. Keep the other leg straight with knee locked. Bring your head toward the knee of the extended leg until it hurts. Hold for 10 elephants. Relax. Repeat for one minute, then do the same exercise with the other leg.

Three • Backover

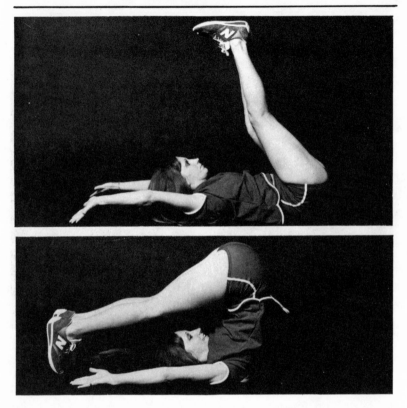

3. The final stretching exercise is the *backover* for the hamstrings and low back. Lie on the floor. Bring straight legs over your head and try to touch the floor with your toes until it hurts. Hold for 10 elephants. Repeat stretch and relax periods for one minute.

Four • Shin Muscles

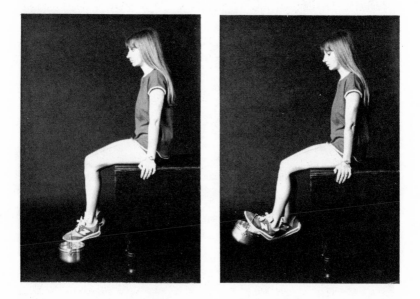

4. The first strengthening exercise is for the *shin muscles.* Sit on a table with the legs hanging down. Put a 3-5 pound weight over the toes. Flex foot at ankle. Hold for six elephants. Relax. Repeat for one minute with each leg.

Five • Quadriceps

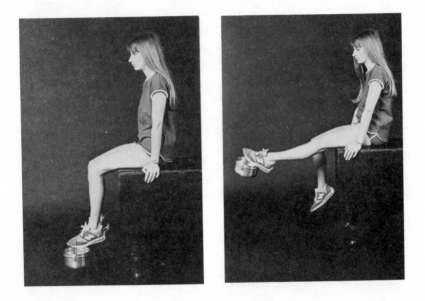

5. The second is for the quadriceps (thigh muscles). Assume the same position with the weight. This time, straighten the leg, locking the knee. Hold for six elephants. Relax. Repeat for one minute; then do the same with the other leg.

Six • Bent-Leg Situp

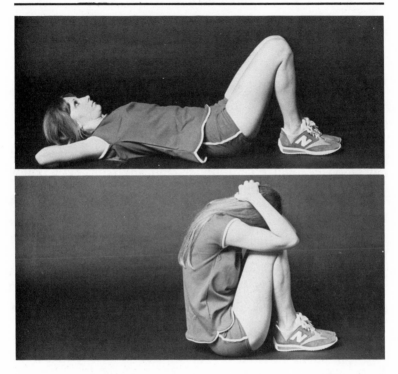

6. The final exercise is the *bent-leg situp.* Lie on the floor with your knees bent and your feet close to your buttocks. Come to a sitting position. Lie back. Repeat until you can't do any more or have reached 20.

6
Learning the Hard Way

Perfect health may seem to be the ideal state of man, and uninterrupted pleasure may be his dream. But pain has positive values, too.

Garrett Tomczak, a runner-writer with philosophical leanings, writes, "If an individual is rational and intelligent, he will soon recognize and understand his pains—you know which ones are warning lights and which are challenges."

He notes that "pain is the transition between different and ever higher levels of consciousness. It can open up profound depths whose existence is not even suspected by the man who goes gaily on his way, untried by pain."

True enough. But perhaps this is a bit too lofty a concept to recognize immediately as being pertinent to running medicine. Dr. George Sheehan, the runners' advisor, is more to the point. He says,"If it weren't for my injuries, I don't know what I'd have to write about in *Runner's World.* I've learned more from my own aches and pains than from my formal medical practice."

"Physician, heal thyself," Nietzsche said a long time ago. And never is a cure so urgent as when the doctor is a runner and he himself is suffering. Dr. Sheehan gets a lot of mileage from his self-treatment. He's forced to find a solution to his own problem. When he finds it, he steps to that higher level of consciousness that Garrett Tomczak describes. Then the doctor gets to tell other runners about his discovery.

This is the advantage of having access to the running press. When most runners are injured, they must suffer in silence. When they discover a personal miracle cure, it generally stays personal. A writer like Dr. Sheehan—or Robert Bahr of *Fitness for Living* or Joe Henderson of *RW*—gets to share his suffering with a mass audience, whether that audience wants to hear it or not.

Those who write about running are just like anyone else who runs. They don't worry much about what they don't have wrong with them. They don't often practice preventive medicine, but only go looking for solutions to problems as pain makes itself felt. Pain demands relief, and in that way is an effective teacher.

The writers, like anyone else, stumble from cure to cure until they find one that works. Then they rush to their typewriters to pound out the success story. The motives are honorable, not self-serving. They want to pass along the lesson so other runners won't have to suffer so much and stumble along so desperately looking for relief.

But not much of the experience seems to sink into a reader until he himself is faced with a similar situation and pain demands that he reread that old article.

Joe Henderson here at *RW* hadn't read the article by Robert Bahr when it first came out in *Fitness for Living* months earlier. It was about exercises, and Henderson was one of those running purists who thought he needed nothing but running. Now Henderson was hurting.

He wrote of an exchange with a doctor. When the doctor bent back the toes on the offending foot, Joe yelped.

"Where does it hurt?" the doctor asked.

"Up here," Henderson said, pointing to his calf.

"Ah ha! Stand up and bend over. See if you can touch your toes."

When Henderson tried, his fingertips stopped high on his shins.

"I think I see what might be wrong with you," the doctor said. "Your calves are unusually strong and tight, even for a runner. You're overdeveloped there from your years of running. Your achilles tendon is like a rubber band that is always stretching to the point of breaking. When you put the slightest extra pull on it, something gives. Sometimes it's the achilles itself, sometimes the calf muscle. In this case, it's the area where the tendon attaches to the heel. Unless you do something about those tight calves, you'll keep having trouble."

The doctor didn't say what exactly to do, except to mention "exercises." That's when Henderson went back and reread Bahr. The magazine editor said in effect that his work gave him a headache and his play made him uptight. Henderson, a magazine editor himself, felt the same way. His writing sent him home with a tension headache two or three nights a week. The doctor told him what running had done to his legs.

Bahr's article said, "When there is no effort to maintain flexibility, tendons and ligaments (as well as muscles) shorten with the passing of time. Occasionally, calcium deposits may build up." Henderson had calcium deposits forming at the points on both feet where the achilles tendons insert into the heel bone, and one of the lumps was inflamed. Bahr had his interest.

One night Bahr had been particularly achy. He couldn't sleep, so he got up to do some relaxing exercises. "I climbed out of bed, sat on the floor and tried to touch my toes," he said. "Even I was astonished. I could not even reach my ankles. Right there and then I devised three stretch exercises for taking the tension out of the body." (See the accompanying photos.)

He mentioned yoga. Henderson had never thought of yoga in connection with running, but now he was in the "I'll-try-anything" stage.

"If yoga exercises do anything," Bahr writes, "they force you to loosen up again. Every position requires you to stretch and loosen a ligament, tendon or muscle you've spent a lifetime tightening." He warned that the exercises must be done "without significant strain, jerking movements or force."

After a couple of months on Bahr's basic three positions, Henderson rushed to his typewriter to pound out a story for RW. He told what a rude shock the beginning had been. Bahr had said, "It works so well it truly amazes me." But Henderson's intial burst of enthusiasm was replaced quickly by frustration with his extreme limitations. He felt much as a beginning distance runner must feel in his first few weeks: eager, then discouraged, then finally determined to push forward at his own rate.

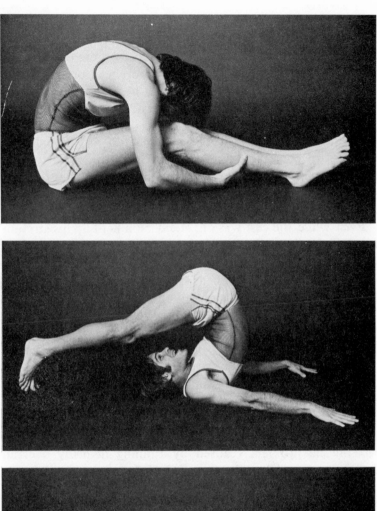

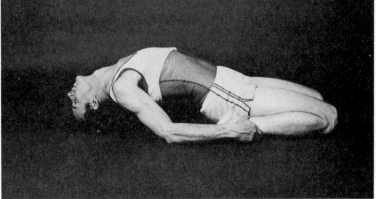

He wrote, "When you're a total novice like I am, victories have to be small ones. After three weeks of everyday stretching, my fingers barely scraped the carpet on the floor on the plough. I grazed my knees with my forehead on the sitting toe-touch (we'll forget for now that there was six inches of daylight under the knees). I felt happy as a jogger must when he gets through his first mile."

The damage to Joe's feet had gone too far, though, for exercises to correct. He needed surgery on one heel to take out a calcium deposit which was irritating an achilles tendon. The doctor said, "It may be as much as a year before you're back to normal."

Even while the cast was on, Henderson kept up his stretching. By this time, he'd added new positions for a total of about ten a day. (Bahr's plus others covered later in this section). The session took 15-20 minutes each evening, or as he put it, "one side of a record album."

As soon as the cast came off, he was running again. Seven months later, he ran a marathon almost as fast as any he'd done before the operation. Both he and the doctor attribute the quicker-than-normal recovery to the stretching.

"I'm sure this is true," Henderson says, "because if I skip even one night of stretching the repaired heel, I'm very stiff there the next morning when I run."

Any other obvious benefits? "I *feel* that I got over a minor calf muscle problem (caused by running in badly overrun shoes) much quicker than usual. I *feel* my running action is smoother, more fluid than ever before. But I can't really prove any of these things."

One thing he can prove is that he's having fewer headaches after days of writing. This has been an unexpected bonus from the stretching. "The exercises drain away tension," Henderson says. "I don't have one headache a month now."

He admits, though, that progress hasn't been startling, and that even after a year of this he still could barely meet Hans Kraus's minimum fitness standard of a simple floor touch.

"It was almost 11 months from the time I started stretching until I first scraped the floor with my fingernails,"

Joe says. "When I did it, I felt almost as happy as when I first broke three hours in the marathon.

"I know this isn't much of a feat, any more than breaking three hours is that impressive. But I was elated just to have come this far, no matter how long it took. If it hadn't been a pleasant kind of exercise in itself, I probably wouldn't have bothered to come."

The pleasant trip began with pain.

References

Part Two

Bahr, Robert. "From the Fitness House." *Fitness for Living,* May-June 1972, pp. 4-6.

Bahr, Robert. "Stretch Those Muscles." *Fitness for Living,* July-August 1972, pp. 65-71.

De Vries, Herbert A. *Physiology of Exercise for Physical Education and Athletics.* Dubuque, Iowa: William C. Brown, Co., 1966.

Falls, H.B.; Wallis E.L.; and Logan, G.A. *Foundations of Conditioning.* New York: Academic Press, 1970.

Henderson, Joe. "The Runner's Final Stretch." *Runner's World,* January 1973, pp. 41-43.

Hittleman, Richard. *Be Young with Yoga.* New York: Paperback Library, 1962.

Hittleman, Richard. *Yoga 28-Day Exercise Plan.* New York: Workman Publishing Co., 1969.

Iyengar, B.K.S. *Light on Yoga.* New York: Schocken Books, 1965.

Jackson, Ian. "The Root of All Training." *Runner's World,* May 1973.

Rawls, Eugene S. *A Handbook of Yoga for Modern Living.* New York: Pyramid Books, 1964.

Ruchpaul, Eva. *Hatha Yoga.* New York: Funk and Wagnalls, 1969.

Tomczak, Garrett. "Is Pain Necessary?" *Runner's World,* April 1973, pp. 20-21.

Recommended Reading

Higdon, Hal. *Beginners Running Guide.* Mountain View, Calif.: World Publications 1978.

The Complete Runner. Mountain View: World Publications. 1974.

III
Yoga for the Runner

7
No Strain, No Pain

The roots of sound stretching techniques go back some 4000 years. Yoga originated in India at least that long ago, and it has come to be an entire life philosophy for those who take it seriously.

Our concern here is only with the physical side of it—the "hatha yoga" practice. The spiritual meditative side is ignored, though this kind of separation is foreign to the yoga way of thinking. The word yoga in sanskrit means "unity," and when mind and body are split much is lost.

May the yogis forgive us for borrowing so shamelessly to suit our own needs. No doubt we've lost sight of the true aim of yoga, which is self-control and self-understanding far beyond anything running can give. Perhaps because Western man is more physical and segmented in his outlook than the Indian, the exercise part of yoga always has received more attention in North America and Europe than have the contemplative features.

Old-line yogis might freeze in their lotus postures if they read how their ancient art has been cheapened on early-morning television shows for overweight housewives and in mass-circulation magazines for over-tensed businessmen (to say nothing of booklets for over-run runners).

Apparently, though, even this fraction of yoga has much to offer. And it has the versatility to offer its values to people who wouldn't any more meditate than bathe in the Ganges. Hatha Yoga has an appeal lacking in other, newer forms of bending and stretching. Hence, the growing popularity.

Richard Hittleman hosts a TV exercise series called "Yoga for Health." His following is so wide that he has had to write five yoga books to satisfy the demand. Hittleman has been a leading translator of yoga principles into the Western way of thinking and exercising. He hasn't compromised the basic integrity of the system. He merely emphasizes what Americans want to hear and do.

Hittleman writes, "Stretching is the key to relieving tension and releasing energy." The yoga *asanas* (postures), in their infinite variety, all concentrate on gently stretching away the forces that make people look and feel uptight.

Yoga isn't like the exercise Westerners have grown up with in school sports. There is none of the strain and pain, sudden movement, exertion or repetition of calisthenics.

"Inherent in most systems of calisthenics," Hittleman says, "is the need to execute many quick repetitions or exercises, huff, puff, perspire and experience general discomfort and fatigue...But meaningful exercise, which I define in terms of *methodical body manipulation,* need contain none of the above.

"Indeed, a yoga session is designed to be a highly pleasurable experience in which the exact opposites are true. That is, the movements are performed in relaxing slow motion with very few repetitions. No strain should ever be felt, and the practice sessions leave you feeling elevated and revitalized, not drained."

There is no place for hurry or for competitive urges in yoga. Save those for the track and road. Yoga above all requires great patience, concentration and control.

Hittleman says, "Remember that you must never strain, jerk or fight to achieve a more extreme position. Just go as far as you can, regardless of where it may be, and have the patience to hold (the posture) as indicated. The 'hold' will gradually impart the elasticity that is needed to accomplish the most extreme positions."

He claims that as long as the demands on the body are moderate but regular, the flexibility to accomplish the extreme positions comes with time. It may be a long time coming, he says, but don't rush. People who hurry in yoga only get hurt. One has to work within his own limitations and progress at his own rate.

Hittlemen's advice here is particularly relevant to tight runners: "It is well to remember that most physical problems have developed over a period of time—months or years. And when attempting to deal with them through natural means, such as yoga, it is unrealistic to expect an immediate solution. If the laws of nature have been abused for prolonged periods, no sudden reversal of the resultant condition can be expected."

Yoga requires no apparatus, no pain, only a little sweat. All it really takes is time, which as it turns out is the hardest thing for a Westerner to give. Yogis, with 40 centuries of tradition backing them, talk as if they have all the time in the world. A busy, impatient runner who's already spending an hour or so a day in sport needs convincing that the extra minutes of yoga are necessary.

8
Yoga for the Runner
Ian Jackson

I used to believe that distance runners were biologically unique, gifted with inborn endurance capacities that an average individual (like myself) could never dream of matching. I used to believe the same things about yoga adepts too—that their incredible flexibility was an inborn trait, something that set them apart from the average.

Now I realize that we all have great endurance capacities lying dormant within the very structure of our tissues, waiting to be tapped. I realize the same thing about flexibility. It is a potential in all of us, and it's waiting to be released. This story tells how the excitement of releasing endurance pushed me to run myself right out of running, and how the excitement of releasing flexibility pushed me, gently, right back in.

I first tried endurance training several years after my mediocre career in college cross-country and track. I didn't think of it as training at the time—it was just aerobic health running, inspired by Dr. Kenneth Cooper's revolutionary book *Aerobics.* But once I had made reasonable progess, I began getting encouragement from competitive runners, and further inspiration from books they recommended to me— books like Joe Henderson's *LSD: The Humane Way to Train,* and Tom Osler's *The Conditioning of Distance Runners.*

These influences gradually revised my belief that I was biologically disqualified from distance running. Eventually they led me to the starting line of my first marathon. And to my very pleasant surprise, they led me all the way to the

Ian Jackson, a frequent contributor to *Runner's World* magazine, is author of *Yoga and The Athlete* (Mountain View, Calif.: World Publications, 1975). He outlined the Eighteen-Week Yoga Plan in the next chapter.

finish line. Although my time was not good, I was elated simply to have finished. The race was so thoroughly enjoyable I decided right there and then that there would be plenty more "next times." Over the next year or so, there were indeed plenty more—with distances ranging from 10 to 50 kilometers. There was also a steady improvement in times and placings, and improvement which kept me constantly surprised and disbelieving. ("The watches must be off." "The course must be short." "Anyone I beat must have had a bad day.")

Finally, however, the disbelief abated. I began to see myself in the role of a competitor more than a health runner—a contender for high places in local races. A few experiences out in front were sufficient. Once I had tasted the blend of fierce, competitive intensity and precise control of power, I was hooked. I wanted more than anything to multiply, to refine, and to expand those peak experiences through ever greater racing achievements.

This new attitude was the beginning of the end for my running. Over the next few months my workouts grew steadily longer and faster. At first I went through a tremendous surge in strength and endurance. At first my dreams of top-class racing seemed to be coming true. But then things started to go wrong. My legs seemed always to be sore and stiff. I went through uncharacteristic mood changes; I felt generally clumsy and uncoordinated. I was often tired from one workout to the next.

I was overtraining, overstressing myself, forcing a slow and inexorable breakdown by pushing myself too hard. As I explained in a *Runner's World* article, I came to realize what I was doing through Hans Selye's brilliant and widely acclaimed book, *The Stress of Life.* Besides helping me understand the problem of excess stress, Selye's book also gave me some excellent advice on what to do about it.

The most important (and least expected) advice dealt with two philosophical issues: (1) the problems of interpersonal relationships and (2) the need for an ultimate goal in life. In the first place, the needless stressors of "fights, frustrations, and insecurities" could be eliminated by living so as to earn the gratitude, rather than the revenge of others. In the second place, the stress of aimlessly drifting through life could be eliminated by adopting the philosophy of "expressing (oneself) fully, according to (one's) own lights."

As Selye points out in his inspiring discussion, adapting wisely to stress "is not easy...It takes much practice and almost constant self-analysis." This kind of effort was the last thing I expected to take on when I first started my running for fitness, but I see it now as a logical development. After all, a superior heart-lung system is wasted in a person crippled by frustrations, hostilities, and anxieties. I agree with Selye—this effort is not easy, but the rewards are abundant. As I practiced his philosophy, I found my life becoming brighter, simpler, more fulfilling, and more meaningful.

As for my running, I simply cut down on the speed and distance, dropped my competitive obsessions, and started enjoying myself again. Almost all the symptoms of overstress dropped away and I felt myself entering into a new mode of balanced, harmonious living.

Undoing the Damage

There was only one remaining problem—my legs seemed to be disintegrating. In several hard races, I had become so completely absorbed in the struggle that the pains in my legs could not penetrate into my awareness until I crossed the finish line and slowed down. The same pattern was repeated on a larger scale now: All the pains that my racing obesession had masked suddenly came to life and clamored for attention.

I had been aware of low-level soreness and tightness for some time, but I was totally unprepared for the interlaced agony that now seized me. Hips, thighs, knees, shins, ankles, feet and especially hamstrings, as if overjoyed to have an opportunity, now began screaming accusations of abuse at me.

I was appalled at this evidence of severe overwork, and amazed that I had been able to suppress the pain for so long. No matter how much I cut down on pace and distance, the pains got worse. My right hamstring was so bad that I thought it must be severely torn or traumatized. Running friends suggested that I might have sciatica.

At this critical period of confusion, I came across the Joe Henderson article on stretching and muscular imbalance, which is described earlier in this book, and I was relieved to find such a simple explanation for my problems. All I had to do now was to add a little stretching to my daily routine—or so I thought, until I actually tried the positions shown in the stretching exercise photos. I failed miserably on all of them. In a half-hour of red-faced, futile struggling I could not even come close to achieving them.

After this humiliation, I wanted nothing more to do with them. The idea of facing that frustrating failure in a daily stretching session didn't appeal to me at all. Rather, I created an ingenious fantasy to soften the sting of defeat. I could easily attain those positions, I told myself, if only I did a few warm-up stretches first. After all, my stiffness was only superficial, like a dried crust of mud on a running shoe. A few good twists and flexes would break up the crust of muscle stiffness as easily as a crust of dried mud.

Yoga was mentioned in the *RW* article, so I decided to consult some yoga books, feeling confident that they would show me the secret. I toured a few used book stores (like many runners, I am a pauper), and returned home with a handful of hatha yoga texts. All I needed now was to find a progressive sequence of stretches to lead quickly and efficiently to the kind of flexibility demonstrated in the photos.

But what a surprise I got when I looked closely into the books I had bought. Although Robert Bahr's positions had looked easy, they had been impossible. The positions in the books did not even look easy. The photos showed dark, intense-looking Indians, "sitting," "standing," or "lying" in extreme pretzel-twisted positions that made Bahr's look like child's play. They were downright discouraging.

Luckily, some of the books in my selection seemed to understand my problem. I found one particularly helpful: Richard Hittleman's *Be Young With Yoga,* a step-by-step, seven-week program in the course of which 20 yoga practices are learned. Another helpful book was Eugene Rawls's *A Handbook of Yoga for Modern Living.*

Although I'd found an ideal introductory program, my problems were far from over. I still entertained delusions about my stiffness. I still thought it was a superficial crust, as easy to break as the dried mud on a shore. I thought I could look forward to complete flexibility by the end of the seven-week program.

Hittleman made it clear that it was foolish to expect such rapid improvement, and I should have realized that a seven-week plan for flexibility was as absurd as a seven-week plan for marathon fitness. However, I convinced myself that I was an exception to the rule, and I started the first week of the program with a determined frontal assault.

The first position was the one that is demonstrated on page 31. Hittleman calls it the "preliminary leg pull." When I tried it the first day, I could barely secure a grip on my shins just below the knee. In this position, my hamstrings and my backbone were stretched about as tightly as possible. But (trying to break through the "crust") I forced my elbows out as far as possible, straining to bring my head down towards my knees. My legs and arms were trembling violently, and the pain was intense. After 10 endless seconds, I released the tension and went on to the other positions, attacking them with the same senseless force.

Hittleman believes that, once you've learned and practiced hatha yoga, "you will find that you will never want to discontinue the exercises." By the end of that first week, however, my legs were more painful than ever, and my whole body ached. Not only did I *want* to discontinue the exercises, I *had* to.

Of course, I was in the wrong, not Hittleman. The frontal, crust-breaking assault that I had been trying was not yoga at all, but a form of self-torture. I reluctantly admitted to myself that my stiffness was far from superficial. It was solidly, deeply rooted. I took a week's layoff to recover. When I started practice again, I read Hittleman's directions with a new respect.

He says you should always stop when "you reach the point

beyond which you can no longer stretch comfortably...for there is never to be any strain in the practice of yoga." This reminded me of Arthur Lydiard's famous principle, "Train, don't strain." Having learned the lesson in running, I should have been more cautious in my approach to yoga. Perhaps all these lessons have to be learned the hard way. Even if I had started stretching gently, sooner or later I would have had to explore straining, if only to discover the difference between practicing too gently and too forcefully.

Learning the distinction between the two is not easy. Even after months of practice I still occasionally suffered soreness after pushing a good stretch into a damaging strain. I can suggest a method that I have found helpful, one that makes you sensitive to muscle tensions. I found it in Eva Ruchpaul's book, *Hatha Yoga*. She recommends what I would call a dynamic stretch, as opposed to Hittleman's static stretch. Instead of holding the yoga pose motionless at the borderline of comfort, Ruchpaul recommends holding it there attentively, waiting for the muscles to relax, and then gently, precisely, taking up the slack.

In the forward bending pose, for instance, you should start by reaching and holding as far down the shins with the hands and as close to the knees with the head as is comfortably possible. Then you should wait, with all your attention concentrated on the stretching muscles, until you sense an easing of the tension. At this point you should widen your elbows and pull down your head so that the slack is taken up. Throughout the duration of the pose, you should keep yourself as focused as possible in your muscle sensations, always balancing the tension right on the edge of comfort.

This method has the advantage of the absorbing fascination of self-exploration. Hittleman's method has the advantage of safety. I use the first when all is going well, and Hittleman's when I am recovering from soreness.

Once I had given up my "crust-breaking" method, and learned correct practice, I began to appreciate just how effective yoga can be. Each session calmed and relaxed me. Some of them, the most perfectly executed of them, were so enjoyable that I would start from the beginning and work my way through all the positions again. Occasionally, I now find myself setting aside a couple of hours on a quieter evening for a session of very slow, very smooth stretches, in which I strive for the utmost in concentration and precision. Can you imagine getting that kind of satisfaction from calisthenics? I can't.

The Major Benefit

What happened as my practice progressed? There were many benefits that I know I would not have experienced with traditional exercises. The most obvious result was that I began to experience the kind of ease in ordinary, everyday activity that I thought was the privilege only of childhood. The changes were gradual and subtle, but their cumulative effect made a great deal of difference.

As I progressed, I realized how profoundly our thoughts and feelings are influenced by simple little consequences of reduced flexibility. For instance, when we can no longer twist our necks and spines, we tend to move our whole bodies to look behind or to the side. Then we tend to resign ourselves with the part of the world that lies straight ahead. The consequences of self-limitations like this are of major importance in the process of physical and psychological aging.

Have you ever watched young children playing on rough ground, running and jumping, with no care whatsoever for the dangers of twists and sprains of the knees and ankles? Better yet, can you conjure up a vivid recollection of yourself when you moved with that same freedom?

I ask these questions because of a remarkable experience I had recently, an experience which dramatically and unexpectedly showed me some of the changes that my yoga practice had brought about. I was hiking in the hills, cautiously making my way down a steep slope, when I stumbled, lost control, and started slipping, sliding, and then running headlong towards the bottom. I thought I was in imminent danger of a sprained ankle or knee, but after just a few steps I realized that there was something radically different in the way I was moving.

As my feet hit the bumps, plunged into the ruts and rolled on the loose stones, they seemed to be flexing and adjusting in a marvellously fluid manner. By the time I reached the bottom of the slope, I realized that I was in no more danger of a sprain than a rubber-limbed child would be. The practice of the lotus pose had made my joints as flexible as they were over 20 years ago. I am probably more flexible right now than I have ever been.

I could mention other minor details, such as being able to sit comfortably erect for hours of reading or writing, and being able to tie my shoelaces without bending my knees and without any tightness in my hamstrings. But rather than giving a catalogue of benefits, I'd like to give the overall impression—the total result of all these little changes in combination. It is best described as a feeling of "weightlessness," a loose, exhilarating, floating feeling of weightlessness.

When I had progressed in hatha yoga for a few weeks, I dropped my running entirely. Frankly, I was tired of running, and I found Yoga just as satisfying, if not more so. I vaguely intended to start running again, but I made no definite plans about it. I might easily have become one of those drop-outs who never runs another step.

Yoga wouldn't let me stop, though. As I got loose and comfortable, as the "weightless" sensation became more constant, I was pushed right back into running. I couldn't help myself. I would be walking to the store, feeling so light and at ease that I would spontaneously break into a run. I just felt an inner, irresistable urge to run, to move rhythmically and smoothly again.

There's something different in the running feeling now, though. It's a subtle difference, but a very pleasant one. Rather than super-efficiency in a stereotyped pattern, outside of which I'm limited by stiffness, I feel competence and ease in a wide range of movements. It's that "weightlessness" again, a natural, loose-swinging freedom. It feels as if running takes far less energy than it used to, and perhaps it actually does. Surely it must take less effort to move limbs well within their range of movement than in a narrow rut which almost defines their range of movement. Of course, I don't know if the change is merely my imagination. We need more widespread experimentation before we can be sure of the effects of flexibility.

Advanced Postures

I stayed on Hittleman's "seven-week" course for five months, until I felt so comfortable with the 20 basic practices that I wanted to learn more. Looking around for a good guide, I found books offering six-, 12-, and 21-week courses, but none of them was exactly what I had in mind.

Finally, I found just the book I was looking for, B.K.S. Iyengar's *Light on Yoga.* Ironically, it was even more imposing than the books I had found so discouraging at the beginning. Now, however, I knew enough about hatha yoga to realize that it would assure me the most rapid progress.

It had a feature similar to Cooper's "point system" in *Aerobics.* All the asanas were given ratings from 1-60, according to the degree of difficulty. When I checked the asanas that I had mastered, expecting to find them in the 20-30 range (after all, I had at first thought them impossible), I was flabbergasted to find that they were rated only 1, 2, 3, or 4 at the most.

Light on Yoga had certainly enlightened me. I now realized that Hittleman's course, although an excellent introduction, was absolutely basic, like a YMCA beginning running program. Iyengar's book was of another order entirely, like having Bill Bowerman or Arthur Lydiard as a next-door neighbor and coach.

Light on Yoga must be the most complete guide to hatha yoga available. It has 602 photos illustrating 200 asanas and 15 pranayama (breath-control) techniques. Each asana is explained in great detail, with very precise instructions about the muscular stretches that should be experienced with correct practice.

Iyengar points out in his introduction that there are eight stages in yoga:

1. *Yama* (universal moral commandments);
2. *Niyama* (self-purification by discipline);

3. *Asana* (positions);
4. *Pranayama* (rhythmic control of the breath);
5. *Pratyahara* (withdrawal and emancipation of the mind from the domination of the senses and exterior objects);
6. *Dharana* (concentration);
7. *Dhyana* (meditation);
8. *Samadhi* (a state of super-consciousness brought about by profound meditation).

"Practice of asanas without the backing of yama and niyama is mere acrobatics," he states, "without the practice of the principles of yama and niyama, which lay down the foundation for building character, there cannot be an integrated personality."

I know most runners will be primarily interested in the physical benefits of the asanas, and will not be disturbed at lifting them out of context. It won't bother them to practice "mere acrobatics" as long as the practice helps their running. However, since I've already referred to Hans Selye's work, which points out that needless stress can be eliminated by following his "philosophy of gratitude," I think I should bring this forward here.

Selye writes, "In an age so largely governed by intellect as ours, it is gratifying to learn that what religions and philosophies have taught as doctrines to guide our conduct is based on scientifically understandable biologic truths."

The biological truths Selye here refers to are the activities of our glandular and nervous systems in response to stress. Yama and niyama are "doctrines to guide our conduct," which assure the optimum functioning of these stress-adaptive systems. Combined with asanas and the other stages of Yoga practice they produce a state of super-consciousness which radically transforms the individual into transcendent wholeness. This state is as available to persistent, disciplined practice as is superior cardiovascular power. Runners who have experienced extraordinary states of consciousness when in really top condition have felt a hint of what this transcendent wholeness is like.

The average modern man is far below his human potential.

His very life style dooms major areas of his body and mind to disuse and decay. A runner is far above the average: He reaches into the very cellular level of his tissues; his daily runs open vast networks of blood vessels to bring more blood, oxygen, and life to every cell. But unless he balances his life, he too dooms major areas of tissue to disuse and decay. A yoga runner learns to give life to his whole body. Daily, patiently, with persistence and determination, he returns to the effort of awakening *all* the tissues of his life—not just heart and lungs, but muscles, tendons, joints, glands, brain and nerves.

Yehudi Menuhin, the internationally famous violinist, is one of Iyengar's pupils. His life and his art were so profoundly transformed by Yoga that he gave Iyengar a ring, inscribed "To my greatest violin teacher." Now, the discipline of a top runner is nothing like the discipline of a violinist, but Yoga is reputed to release inherent potential so effectively that it produces excellence in any endeavor.

As far as we know, few runners, if any, practice yoga. It's interesting to speculate what would have happened if a great running talent had come under Iyengar's tutelage. Perhaps he'd have a ring inscribed "To my greatest coach."

In his foreword to *Light on Yoga*, Menuhin offers an image of yoga that should appeal to runners, devoted as they are to a spartan, simple, individual quest for excellence: "Yoga, as practiced by Mr. Iyengar, is the dedicated votive offering of a man who brings himself to the altar, alone and clean in body and mind, focused in attention and will, offering in simplicity and innocence not a burnt sacrifice, but simply himself raised to his own highest potential."

Application to Running

Of course, yoga will be for you exactly what you make it. If this holistic view of its meaning does not appeal to you you can still benefit greatly from the "mere acrobatics" of the asanas. These positions, developed and tested over several thousand years, constitute the most sophisticated and comprehensive system of body culture ever known.

The asanas I've chosen here are straight from *Light on*

Yoga. If you're familiar with the basic asanas described in the popular books, you'll notice that several of them are missing. That's because Iyengar's course (which covers 300 weeks—almost six years!) is designed for people who are seriously interested in the science. The asanas are given in an order corresponding to the optimum sequence of development of the body. They are far more strenuous than the popular asanas, and the advanced poses demand and develop exceptional strength. I mention this to dispel the widespread notion that yoga is a discipline for flexibility alone.

Coincidentally, the asanas ideal as starters for runners—the standing asanas—are emphasized at the beginning of the course. As Iyengar points out, "mastery of the standing poses prepares the pupil for the advanced poses in forward bending involve intense hamstring stretches, so these preparatory poses are excellent ways of countering hamstring tightness.

You might think that the advanced poses will be of no value to you, but I think this is a mistaken view. When we're at the very beginning of the trail to fitness, we might find alternate walking and slow running valuable, but once we're in shape, they are a waste of time. The same principle holds in the practice of yoga.

As Iyengar says, "All these intricate and difficult postures bring results quicker than the simpler ones. When the body becomes more pliable, the simple poses will have little or no effect. The wise will therefore discard them and practice the intricate poses just as the scholar will not repeat the alphabet daily."

The asanas which follow are only the alphabet, and yet you'll probably find them far from easy. Don't be discouraged. No matter how stiff you find yourself to be in the beginning, flexibility will reward regular practice in yoga as surely as endurance rewards regular running. If you practice in the morning, the asanas will be harder because your body will be stiff from the night's sleep. If you practice in the evening, they are easiest, but you might find it more difficult to summon the necessary will and concentration. If it's more convenient for you, the practice can be broken into two or three periods per day.

Experiment with the asanas before and after running, and you'll have an unforgettable demonstration of just how stiff a run can leave you. You'll also be able to work out a convenient sequence to stretch your hamstrings at the end of each run. At the moment, the only asana I do after running is a forward bending one, in which I bend over slowly, letting my arms hang down, and then wait for the weight of my trunk to stretch out my hamstrings until I can comfortably rest my palms flat on the ground beside my feet. This usually takes from two to three minutes so I don't start until my breathing is slow. I put in this brief pause because I think (I don't know for a fact) that this prolonged inversion of the trunk should wait for the return of normal circulation.

I wish I could give more specific advice on the application of yoga to running. Our research has shown that there has been very little work, formal or informal, in this area. This outline is only a starting point for further exploration. We would appreciate any comments you have.

9
Eighteen-Week Yoga Plan
Ian Jackson

I have selected the asanas that seem to me to be excellent for runners. Since I am a beginner, my range of choice is severely limited. There are several advanced poses that Iyengar specifically recommends for runners. About one of these, *hanumanasana,* he writes, "This pose helps to cure sciatia and other defects of the legs...and if practiced regularly is recommended for runners. It relaxes and strengthens the abductor muscles of the thighs." The only problem is, the pose has a difficulty rating of 36, so I cannot demonstrate it for you. It's the kind of thing we can keep in mind for later, when these basic positions have long ago been discarded for more intense stretches.

The sequence suggested here should be patiently observed. The time to be spent on each section is a *minimum.* If you desire, you can spend months rather than weeks. You don't have to achieve the final positions of one section before going on to the next, but you should not move on until you feel reasonably comfortable and competent.

You'll notice the sanskrit names of the poses. I do this as a reminder that hatha yoga is radically different from the forms of exercise that we are familiar with. I find that repeating the sanskrit names of the poses before doing them helps to get me in the right frame of mind. My pronunciation is probably all wrong, and I often have to refer back to the book to check myself, but (for me at least) this little ritual is a transition to concentrated attention.

You'll probably find yourself very stiff and sore in the beginning. I think it takes a few painful experiences to learn a healthy respect for these powerful stretches, so you should look upon your early problems as a helpful part of your progress. Don't hesitate to take a few days off whenever you overdo things. It might even be a good idea at first to take a day off each week. I find that an occasional day of doing only the easiest poses seems to bring faster progress.

You'll find the "alphabet" on the following pages. Why not start right now? Stay on each section for at least three weeks. You should never feel you are taking on more than you can handle. If you practice regularly and patiently, you'll amaze yourself. In a few months time, you'll find it hard to believe that these asanas once seemed difficult.

> **Section I**—asanas 1 through 7
> **Section II**—asanas 1 through 9
> **Section III**—asanas 1 through 12
> **Section IV**—asanas 1 through 14
> **Section V**—asanas 1 through 15
> **Section VI**—asanas 1 through 18

Note: although these pictures are good guides, they should not be taken as perfected postures. There are numerous ways to approach each posture, and each time the final pose may be slightly different. Your own body will vary the pose also. The best guide is a well-trained teacher.

1 Triangle Pose DIFFICULTY LEVEL 3

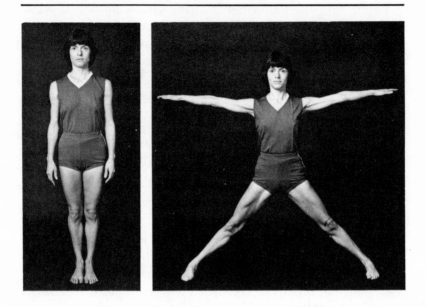

A. All standing postures begin in **Tadasana,** the moun-tain. Stand with toes touch-ing, heels apart about one inch. The kneecaps are pulled up by tightening the thighs. The spine is as long and as straight as possible. The neck is straight.

B. Jump so that feet land about 3-3½ feet apart, arms straight out from the shoul-ders, palms down.

Benefits: This posture tones the leg muscles by stretching the calves and hamstrings. It also strengthens the ankles, removes stiffness in the hips, and develops the chest.

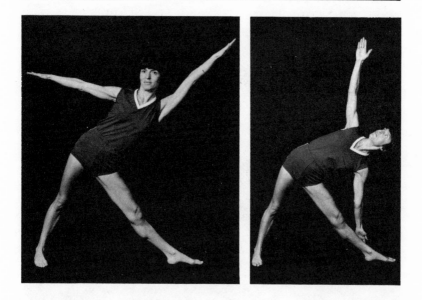

C. Turn left foot 90 degrees to the left, right foot 60 degrees to left. Exhale. Bend at the hip socket and stretch out to the left. Keep the sides of the body long. Knees are locked by pulling up kneecaps.

D. Place left hand on leg. Stretch right arm up in line with left. Twist the body so that the left ribcage comes forward and the right ribcage moves back. Turn head and gaze at the right thumb.

Hold position 30-60 seconds, breathing deeply and evenly. On inhalation, return to upright position **(B)**. Then jump to standing position **(A)**. Repeat exercise on right side.

2 Side Stretch DIFFICULTY LEVEL 4

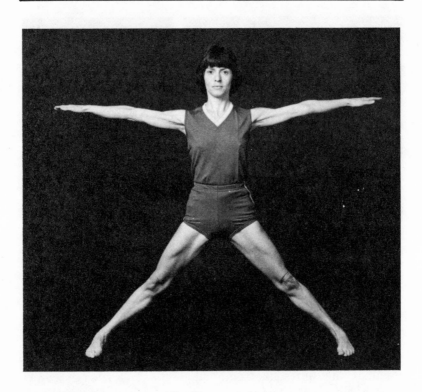

A. Begin in **Tadasana (1A).** Inhale and jump the legs 4-4½ feet apart, arms extended straight out from shoulders, palms down. Turn left foot 90 degrees to left, right foot slightly to left.

Benefits: This pose strengthens and stretches ankles, knees and thighs, particularly works on the calves and thighs.

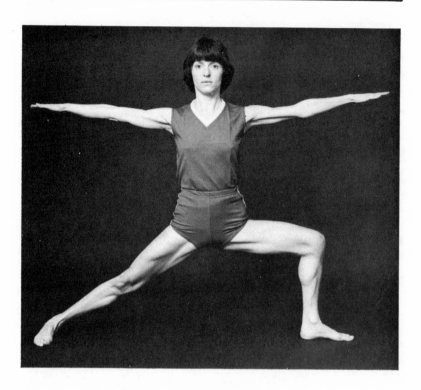

B. As you keep the torso straight, and the right heel on the floor, bend the left leg to form a right angle, thigh parallel to floor.

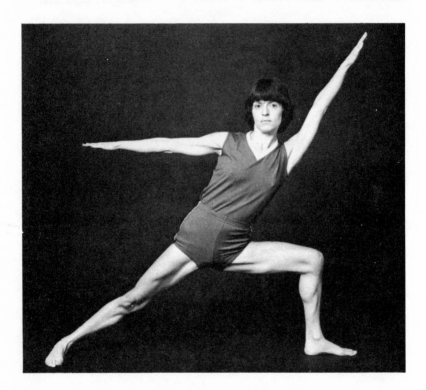

C. Bending at the hips,
stretch the left side out on
the left thigh.

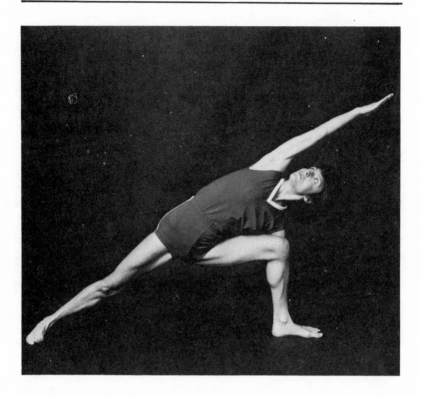

D. Place left hand on floor alongside left foot. Armpit touches outer side of knee. Stretch and straighten right arm over right ear. Keep eyes on right elbow. Move right arm to left keeping both heels on the floor. Stretch so the skin is pulled tight.

Hold position 30-60 seconds, breathing deeply and evenly. Come up from pose with inhalation. Repeat on other side.

3   Fencer's Pose (I) DIFFICULTY LEVEL 3

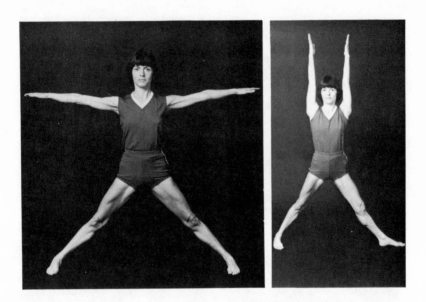

A. Begin in Tadasana **(1A).** Jump the legs 4-4½ feet apart **(2A).**

B. Turn left foot 90 degrees to left, turn right foot slightly to left. Stretch arms above head, palms in, your shoulders down.

Benefits: Here again the legs are being stretched and strengthened. The forward leg is being stretched particularly in the Achilles. The backward leg lengthens in the calf and in the front of the groin.

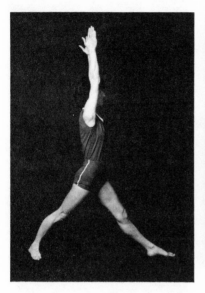 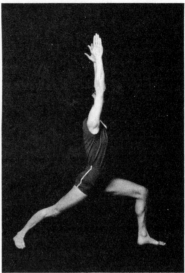

C. Exhale and turn to left. Keep the knees locked by tightening the thighs. Keeping the spine long, bring the right side forward enough to face in same direction as left foot.

D. Bend the left knee to form a right angle. The bent knee is in line with the heel. Keep the right heel on the floor. Stretch spine and arms. Lift head and gaze at palms.

Hold position **(D)** 30-60 seconds, with normal breathing. Exhale. Return to starting position. Repeat on other side.

4 Fencer's Pose (II) DIFFICULTY LEVEL 1

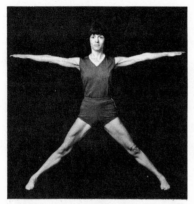

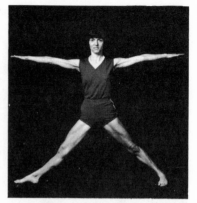

A. Legs 4-4½ feet apart. **(2A).** Stretch arms straight out.

B. Turn right foot 90 degrees to right and left foot slightly to right.

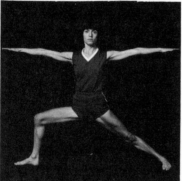

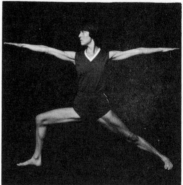

C. While keeping the torso straight, bend the right knee to form a right angle. Stretch left leg, tighten knee, making certain the outer edge of the foot is on the floor.

D. Exhale. Stretch arms as if two people are pulling them in opposite directions. Turn head and gaze at right hand.

Hold position **(D)** 20-30 seconds with normal breathing. Exhale. Return to starting position. Repeat on other side.

Benefits: This pose gives shape to the legs and increases strength. It not only stretches the legs but helps to relieve cramps in the calf and thigh muscles.

5   Intense Side Stretch DIFFICULTY LEVEL 5

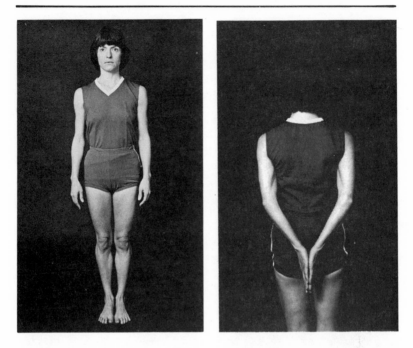

A. Begin in **Tadasana.**   **B.** Bring the palms up together behind the back.

Benefits: This posture relieves stiffness in the legs and hip muscles and gives greater flexibility to the hip joints and spine. Done correctly it also corrects round and drooping shoulders.

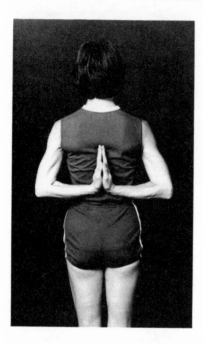 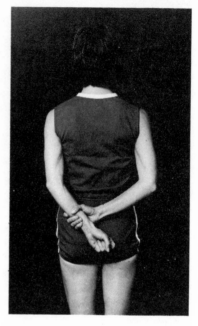

C. Twist the arms, bringing fingers up between shoulder blades. Press the palms flat against each other.

D. Or, if you find B impossible, hold one wrist with the other hand.

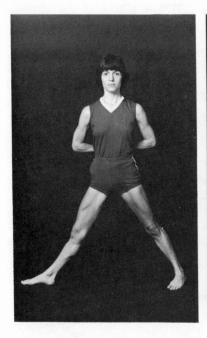 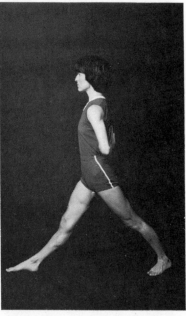

E. Exhale, jump the legs apart 3-3½ feet. Turn right foot 90 degrees to right and left foot 75-80 degrees to right.

F. Inhale and turn trunk to right. Tighten the buttocks to keep the spine long. Bring the left side forward to face in same direction as right foot. Keep both legs straight and tightened at knee.

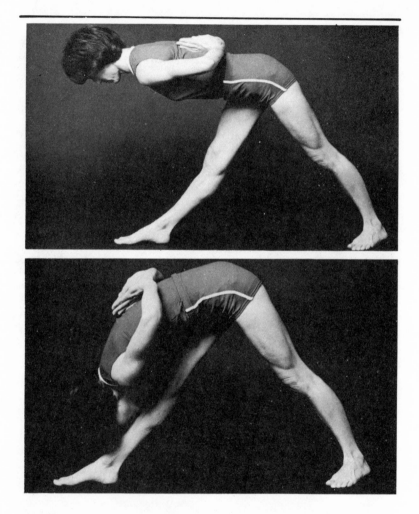

G. Exhale. Keeping both heels on floor, bend forward at the hips with the back straight. Bring the torso parallel to the floor and hold for a couple of breaths.

H. Exhale and bend lower, trying to rest the forehead on the lower leg. Keep both knees tight. Inhale. Straighten. Repeat on other side.

6 Shoulder Stand DIFFICULTY LEVEL 2

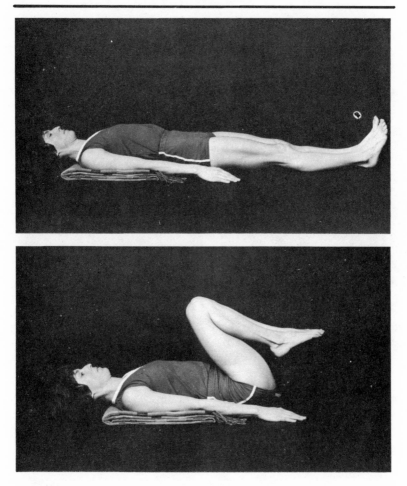

A. Place a folded towel (carpet or mat) under shoulders so that the shoulders are elevated. The head is on the floor. Lie on back. Stretch legs, tighten knees. Hands, palms down, by side of legs.

B. Exhale. Bend the knees, bring thighs up to rest on stomach.

Caution: People with high blood pressure should not do this pose without advise from a teacher.

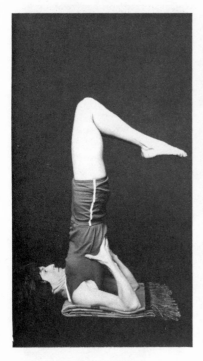 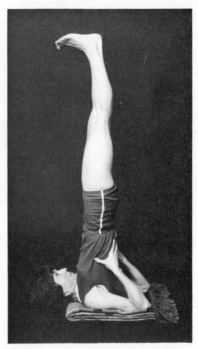

C. Exhale, raise knees up. Press the hands into the back and move the trunk to a vertical position. Bring the elbows toward each other for stronger support.

D. Exhale and stretch legs straight up. As the trunk becomes more vertical, the hands move toward the floor. Tighten knees and buttocks, make the torso as straight as possible.

Hold position **(D)** 5 minutes with even breathing.

Benefits: The shoulder stand is one of the most beneficial poses in yoga. Because it reverses the effects of gravity much of the body is revitalized. The pose stimulates the thyroid and parathyroid particularly. An added supply of blood circulates into the head and the upper body. The shoulder stand is known as the pose of relaxation and will calm the nerves while refreshing the body.

7   The Plough DIFFICULTY LEVEL 4

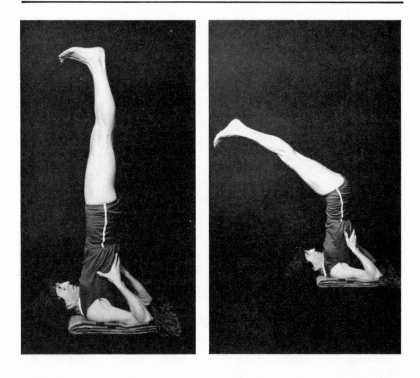

A. Start with the shoulder stand.

B. Keep the torso straight, lower the legs over the head. The feet are arched back, as though standing on them.

Benefits: Besides the internal circulatory effects of being upside down, this posture particularly benefits runners, as it stretches the hamstrings and brings mobility to the back, neck and shoulders.

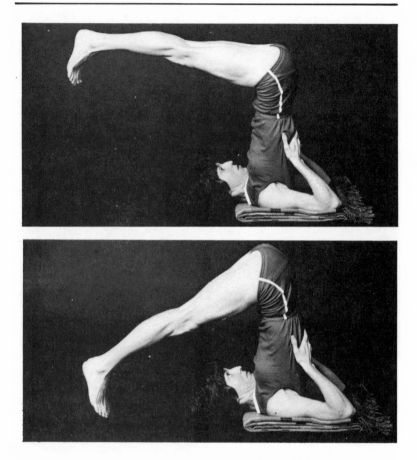

C. This posture stretches the entire back side of the body. If there is difficulty in getting the feet to the floor with the back straight, then place a chair behind the head and rest the toes on it.

D. If possible, continue to lower the feet to the floor. The kneecaps are tight, the buttocks high.

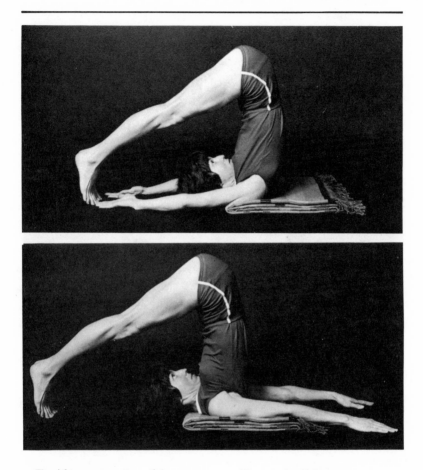

E. Alternate to this arm position, and then . . .   **F.** . . . to this one.

Hold position **(D)** 1-5 minutes with normal breathing.

8   Twisted Triangle DIFFICULTY LEVEL 5

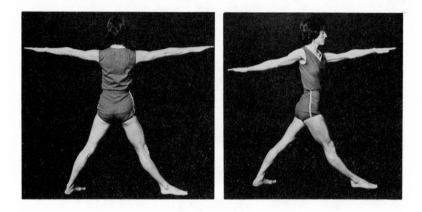

A. Legs 3-3½ feet apart. Arms extended straight out from shoulders, palms down. Turn right foot 90 degrees to right, left foot 60 degrees to left.

B. Exhale. Rotate body to right. Keep left heel on floor and bring left side of body forward to face direction of right foot.

Benefits: This posture stretches and strengthens the thigh, calf, and hamstring muscles. The blood supply is increased in the lower spine bringing health to that area. The hip muscles are strengthened.

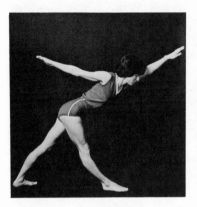

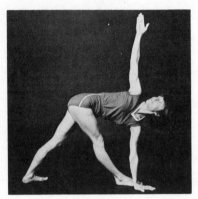

C. Exhale. With the knee-caps pulled up tightly, bend at the hips and stretch the left side forward. Keep both sides of the torso straight.

D. Place the left hand on the floor near the outer side of the right foot. Stretch the right arm up and gaze at the thumb. Open the chest.

Hold position **(D)** 30 seconds with normal breathing. Inhale. Lift palm from floor, return to starting position. Rest if necessary. Repeat on other side.

9 Hanging Stretch DIFFICULTY LEVEL 4

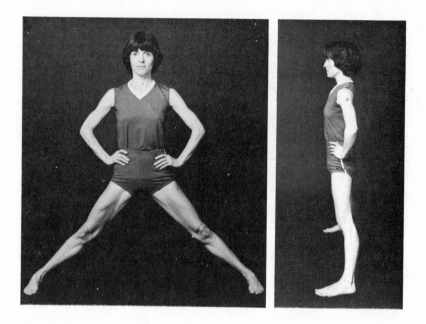

A. Inhale. Place hands on waist. Legs 4½-5 feet apart. Tighten legs by drawing up kneecaps. Lift arches and keep outer edges of the feet on the floor.

B. Same pose, side view.

Benefits: The hamstrings are stretched and the abductor muscles are fully developed. Blood flows to the trunk and upper body, increasing digestive health particularly.

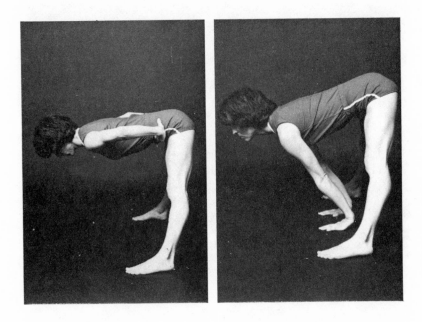

C. Exhale. Bend at hips and bring torso to right angle. Lengthen the spine and try to lift the sitting bones up.

D. Exhale. Place palms on floor between feet and in line with shoulders. Inhale. Raise head up, trying to make back concave.

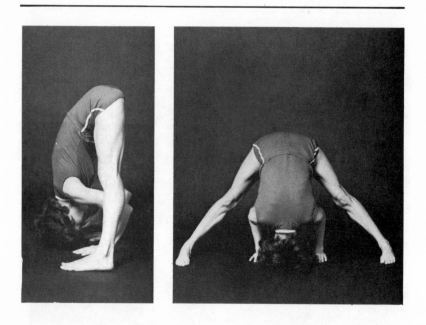

E. Exhale. Bend elbows. Extend trunk down so that crown of head rests on floor keeping body weight on legs.

F. This is how pose looks from front.

Hold position **(F)** 30 seconds, breathing deeply and easily. Inhale. Raise head, straighten arms: Try to make back concave. Inhale. With knees tight and back straight, lift torso to standing position.

10 Leg Lift DIFFICULTY LEVEL 1

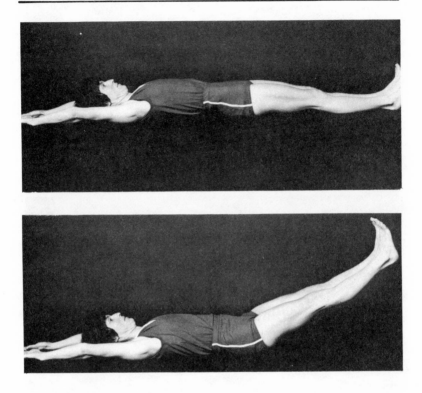

A. Lie flat on back. Make the back long with the waist as close to the floor as possible. Legs stretched out and tightened at knees. Arms stretched straight over head.

B. Exhale. Raise legs to 30-degree angle. With lower back on the floor, hold for 15-20 seconds with normal breathing.

When doing leg lifts, it is important to keep the back on the floor. This way the stomach lifts the legs. If the back lifts off the floor, immediately bend the legs and come out of the pose. Work one leg at a time until abdominal strength can support the legs.

Benefits: This posture strengthens the stomach and back.

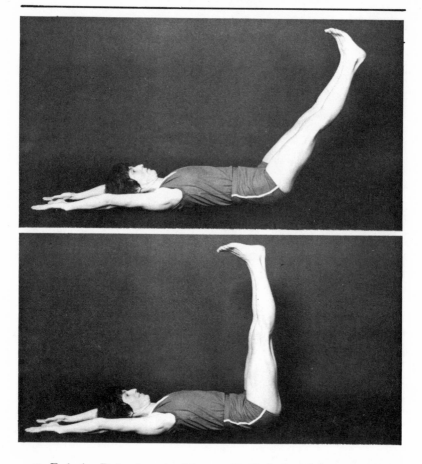

C. Exhale. Raise legs to 60-degree angle. With back on the floor, hold for 15-20 seconds with normal breathing.

D. Exhale. Move the legs to perpendicular. Hold 30-60 seconds with normal breathing. Exhale and lower the legs slowly to the floor and relax. When strength has been acquired lower legs with holds at 60 and 30 degrees. Repeat 3-4 times.

11 The Rowboat DIFFICULTY LEVEL 2

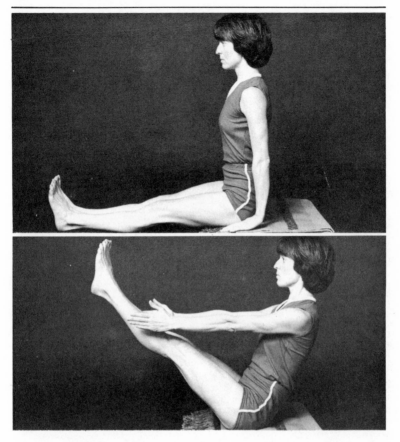

A. Sit on the floor. Legs straight, knees tightened and Palms by hips, with fingers pointing forward. Back as erect as possible.

Hold (**B**) 30 seconds with normal breathing. Exhale. Lower hands, then legs. Relax by lying on back.

B. Exhale. Lean the trunk slightly back and at same time raise legs from floor, keeping them tight. Balance on buttocks, legs at 60-65 degree angle. The back is straight and the feet are slightly higher than the top of the head. Stretch arms out parallel to floor, palms facing each other.

Benefits: Both this pose and **12. The Canoe** work to strengthen the lower back and abdomen.

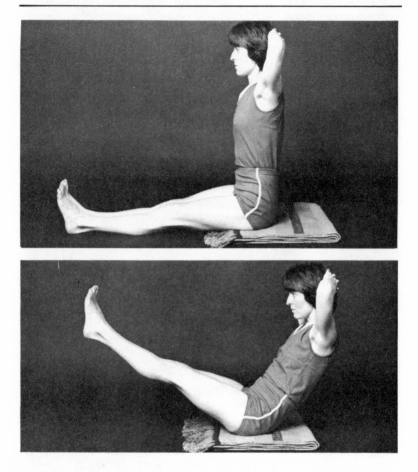

12   The Canoe DIFFICULTY LEVEL 2

A. Sit on the floor. Legs straight, knees tightened. The back as erect as possible. Interlace fingers behind head.

B. Exhale. Recline trunk back and raise legs, keeping knees tightened. The back rounds. Keep legs at 30-35 degree angle, toes level with eyes.

Hold position **(B)** 20-30 seconds with normal breathing. Lower the trunk and legs. Relax by lying on back.

13   Stork Stretch DIFFICULTY LEVEL 5

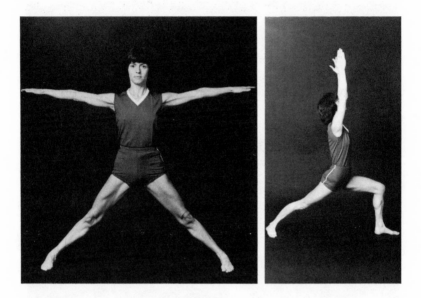

A. Legs 4-4½ feet apart. Stretch arms above head. Turn left foot 90 degrees to left, right foot slightly to right.

B. Bend right knee to form right angle.

Benefits: This pose is particularly recommended for runners because it increases agility and vigor.

VIRABHDRASANA III

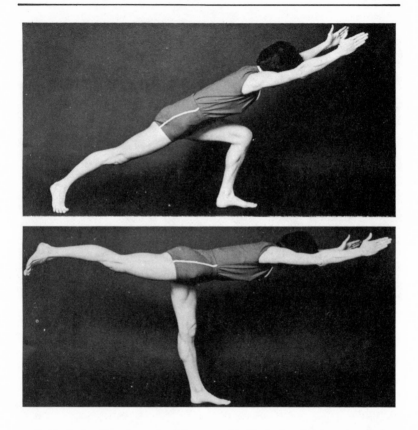

C. Exhale. Bend at the hips and stretch the chest forward to rest on left thigh. Take two breaths.

D. Exhale, lifting back leg by swinging body slightly forward. Straighten support leg and tighten knee. This leg should be perpendicular to floor. Turn the right leg inwards so that leg, body and extended arms are parallel to floor.

Hold position **(D)** 20-30 seconds with deep, even breathing. Repeat on other side.

14   Half-Moon Pose DIFFICULTY LEVEL 5

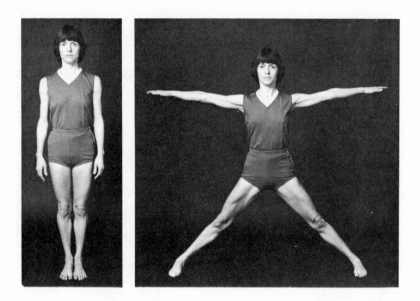

A. Begin in **Tadasana**.

B. Jump so that feet land about one yard apart, arms straight out from shoulders, palms down.

Benefits: This posture tones the lower spine and the nerves connected to the legs. It particularly strengthens the knees.

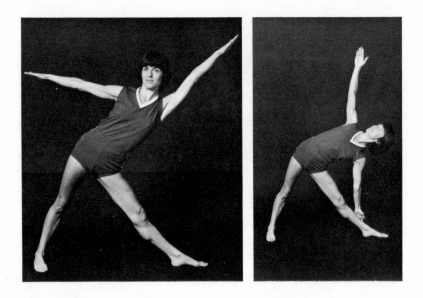

C. Turn left foot 90 degrees to the left; right foot 60 degrees to left. Exhale. Bend at the hip socket and stretch out to the left. Keep the sides of the body long. Knees are locked by pulling up kneecaps.

D. Place left hand on leg. Stretch right arm up in line with left. Twist the body so that the left ribcage comes forward and right ribcage moves back. Turn head and gaze at right thumb.

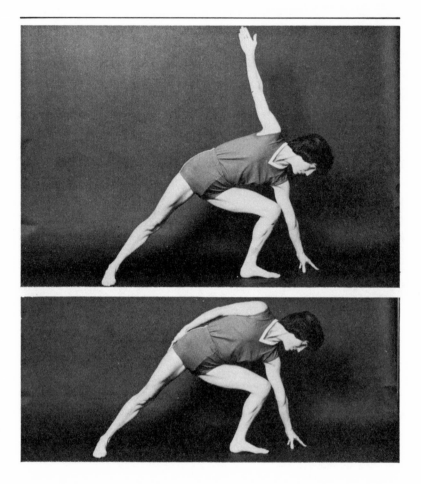

E. After attaining the **Triangle Pose** on the left side, turn head and look down. Bend the left knee and place the finger tips of the left hand one foot away and a little behind the left foot.

F. Bring the right arm down and place it on the right side. Keep the body sideways as much as possible. Hold this position, taking two breaths.

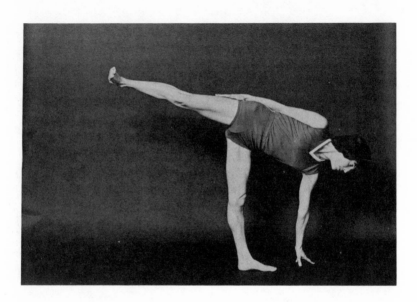

G. Exhale. As the left leg straightens, draw the right toe in toward the body so that body weight is over left leg, then lift right leg laterally until it aligns with the right side of the body.

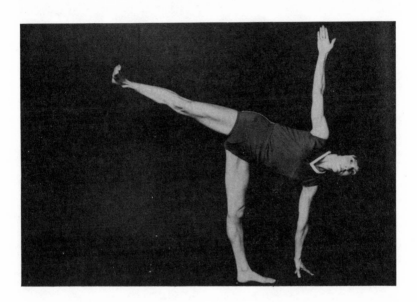

H. When balance is secure, lift right arm straight up. The body is sideways as much as possible with the entire right side up. Both sides of the body are long. Bear the body weight on the left foot and hip, using the left hand only to aid balance. As in all standing postures the thighs are tightened, pulling the kneecaps up.

Hold position **(H)** 20-30 seconds, breathing deeply and easily.

Place right foot to floor, return to the **Triangle Pose, then stand. Repeat**

15 Twisted Side Stretch DIFFICULTY LEVEL 8

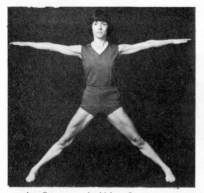 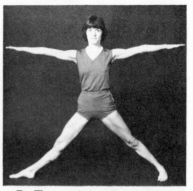

A. Legs 4-4½ feet apart **(2A).** Stretch arms straight out.

B. Turn right foot 90 degrees to right, left foot slightly to right.

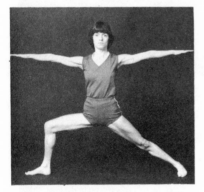 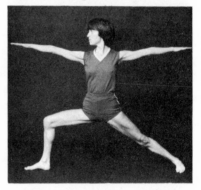

C. Keep the torso straight, and bend the right knee to form a right angle. Stretch left leg, tighten knee, making sure the outer edge of the foot is on the floor.

D. Exhale. Stretch arms as if two people are pulling them in opposite directions. Turn head and gaze at right hand.

Benefits: This posture continues to stretch the legs more deeply, particularly on the lower leg and achilles. The twist in the spine keeps the back young and elastic. All standing postures tone the abdominal area, and this pose especially aids in digestion.

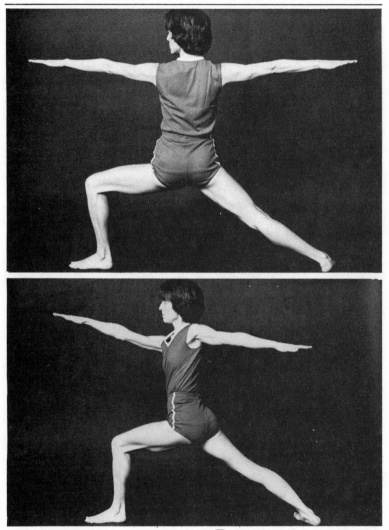

E. Legs 4-4½ feet apart. Arms extended straight out from shoulders, palms down. Turn left foot 90 degrees to left, right foot 60 degrees to left. Bend left leg to form right angle, thigh parallel to floor.

F. Exhale. Rotate the torso and right leg so as to bring the right arm over the left knee. Right leg stretched with kneecap tight and heel on the floor.

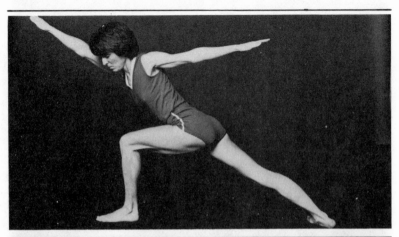

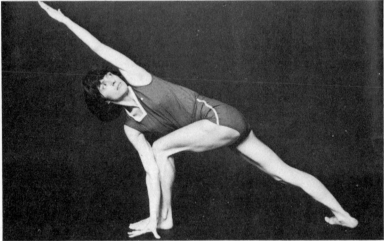

G. Exhale. Bend at the left hip and stretch the right side forward. The spine is long with no bending at the sides.

H. Bring the right arm over knee. Rest right armpit on outer side of knee. Place fingers on floor by outer side of foot. Bring left arm over right ear, head turns up. Give the spine a spiral twist by stretching the entire body from right heel to left finger tips.

16 Hamstring Stretch DIFFICULTY LEVEL 3

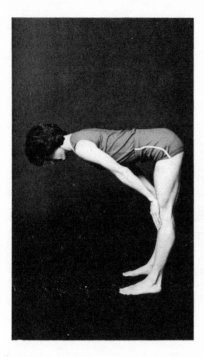 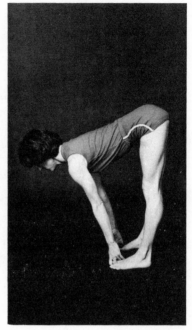

A. Stand with the feet a foot apart. Exhale. Bend at the hips and come forward to 90 degrees. Keep the kneecaps pulled up. Hold for a couple of breaths working to make the spine longer. The sitting bones lift higher.

B. Exhale. Bend forward again and grasp the big toes between thumbs and first two fingers, palms facing each other. (Hold onto legs if hands can't reach the toes yet.) Lift the head up and make the back as concave as possible. Hold for a couple of breaths while working to lengthen spine.

Benefits: This pose achieves greater flexibility on the entire back of the body. The stretch will be beneficial to the hamstring particularly.

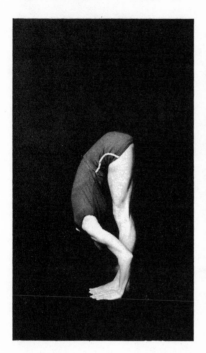
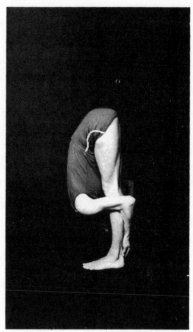

C. Exhale and bend elbows out. Bring the head and torso as low as possible, holding for about 20 seconds. When more advanced, the hands can be placed next to the feet as shown.

D. To work the pose more deeply, place the forearms behind the calves. Press the sitting bones higher, away from the heels, and with each breath stretch the spine so that the head comes closer to the feet. Inhale and stand.

17 Dog Poses DIFFICULTY LEVEL 1 AND 5

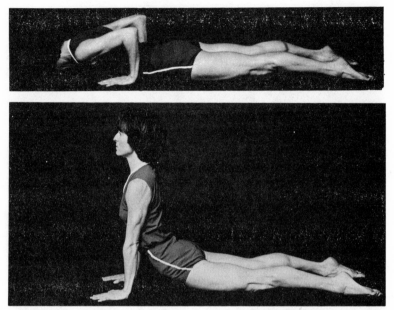

A. Lie on stomach, forehead on floor. Feet one foot apart, toes pointed, knees locked and facing floor. Place palms next to chest, fingers pointing to the head. Elbows in next to body.

B. Inhale. Tighten the buttocks (important, because this protects the lower back), and the knees, as the arms are straightened. The knees are slightly off the floor, the shoulders are low, away from the ears. Open the chest, relax the abdomen area, look straight forward. Hold for a breath or two.

Benefits: This pose is particularly beneficial for runners. The first part keeps the back elastic. The second part relieves pain and stiffness in the heels, strengthens the ankles, and stretches the entire back of the leg. The posture removes fatigue and brings back lost energy so is especially good after running. With frequent practice it will develop speed and lightness in the legs.

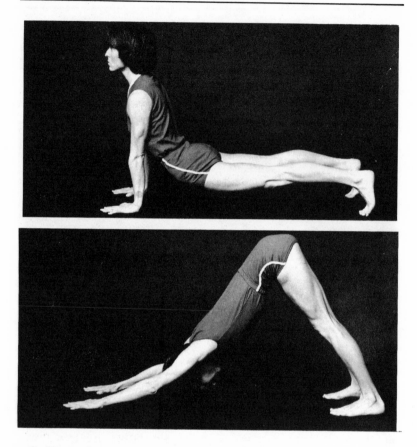

C. Turn the toes up toward the knees. Keep the knees tight and stretch the heels back while continuing to open the chest.

D. Stay high up on the toes, push the buttocks up and back. Straighten the legs. Stay up on toes and tilt the lower back so the sitting bones face directly up. This helps to hollow out the back. Keep this angle in the back and slowly work the heels to the floor. Hold and breathe deeply and evenly.

18 The Camel DIFFICULTY LEVEL 3

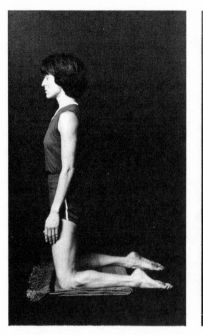 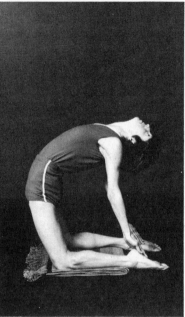

A. Kneel on the floor, thighs and feet one foot apart, toes pointing back. Exhale. Lean back slightly and place the left palm on left heel. Then place right palm on right heel.

B. Press the feet with the palms, contract the buttocks, and drop the head back. Push the spine towards the thighs. Hold for half a minute with normal breathing. Release the hands one at a time. Sit on the floor and relax.

Benefits: Besides opening the chest and strengthening the back, this pose is particularly good for runners because it stretches the front of the thighs, the front of the hips, and helps to keep the knees free of injury.

IV
Weight Training for Men

10

Extremes of Fitness
Charles Palmer

I don't recall just what inspired me to send away for a
set of barbells when I was 14. But I know it wasn't the sight
of some over-upholstered body-builder on the back of a
comic book, daring me to be a man. Maybe it was the recollection of the rather lean weight lifter on a TV newsreel
years earlier, hoisting an enormous weight overhead in two
quick, casual motions, only to momentarily lose control
of the weight and step out from under it with equally casual
aplomb, the weight crashing to the platform, the lifter
dancing back, unhurt, undaunted.

After two years of using that first set of weights in my
basement, hoping to get strong enough to make the first
strain in wrestling, I went to a gym instructor to get a specific wrestling program. He told me I'd have a better chance to
excel in Olympic lifting than wrestling because of my heavy
bone structure and the good strength in my legs and back.
("Olympic" lifting refers to a *style* of lifting, not to the
competition every four years that is most people's only
glimpse at this sport.) I believed him.

The recollection of the flashy performer on the newsreel
from my childhood became more vivid as I plunged into the
"iron game." After a couple of years of specializing on this
most unsung sport. I reached a point where I could clean
(shoulder) and nearly jerk (put overhead to arms' length)
290 pounds. This was still more than 100 pounds below the
world record in my weight class (165 pounds), but I was
considered promising.

Then I learned that anyone who lifted much better than

Chuck Palmer has been to the apparent extremes of athletics—from
competitive weight lifting to competitive running. In the next two
chapters he explodes some of the myths associated with weight lifting
and outlines a weight program for runners.

that was taking "The Pill"—anabolic steroids. This is a drug developed to spur growth in youngsters who are growing too slowly and to aid protein assimilation in older people who have one foot in the grave and the other on a banana peel. When I found that lifters had been using steroids for nearly 10 years (with shot put, discus and hammer men following soon after), I decided to return to training for fitness and feeling good (it always felt good to lift weights) instead of becoming a private drug experiment. This I did on a rather irregular basis while teaching a course in basic weight training at the college I was attending.

Partly in search of a different kind of fitness, partly because of lucid articles in *Playboy* and the *New York Times,* I began to run around a nearby golf course. I became an unconscious "fun-runner" before anyone could tell me that my 165 pounds (even if I was still rather muscular) when carried on a 5'7" frame would limit performance over any distance longer than a quarter-mile.

When I ran across *Runner's World,* it was a joy to find kindred souls who actually came out with a magazine about all this—a *monthly* yet! Finding out I had a ponderal index of 12.2 (this is a relationship of height to weight; most good distance runners are above 13) was somehow less insulting than the necessity to ingest steroids, and within a few months I decided I wanted to follow the original inspiration and run a marathon myself.

And a strange thing happened. After fighting my way up to 50 miles a week, seemingly getting the "injury of the month" almost in sequence with the articles in *RW*, I found that if I combined just a few stretching exercises (chosen to condition the special muscles which were affected by running), I could increase my mileage and not be burdened by that nasty trail of little injuries—aches and pains that served as excuses to avoid training, or, worse, made me doubt the value of running itself.

11
Lifting the Mythology
Charles Palmer

When asked to prepare the strength-training section of this book, I was at first flattered and then apprehensive. Hadn't it all been said before, and better? John Jesse's excellent *Strength, Power and Muscular Endurance for Runners and Hurdlers* came to mind, and I ran across a number of other excellent works as I dug into the literature of strength training for athletes.

Then it occurred to me that beyond a description of a few basic exercises, what was needed most was a general "demythologizing" of the many popular notions surrounding weight lifting. Judging from the reaction I had received in the past when I was exposed as "one of those weight lifters" and the overabundance of pernicious falsehoods circulating about strength training, it was something that was much more urgently needed than merely another description of exercises. The magnitude of my personal ire about the situation, coupled with my experience as a lifter, qualified me for the task.

First, we should distinguish between body-builders, Olympic- and power-lifters, and weight-trained athletes:

• Body-builders seek to maximize muscular size and definition through training that yields strength only as a by-product.

• Olympic-lifters train to maximize their performance on two lifts: the snatch (one motion from the floor to arms' length overhead) and the clean and jerk (one motion to the shoulders, followed by a jerk to arms' length overhead). A third lift, the press, was dropped after the 1972 Olympics because the style of its performance had grown progressively looser through the years, and it was impossible to judge consistently.

Power-lifters specialize in raw strength in the performance

of the deep knee-bend, bench press, and dead-lift and are not overly concerned with style, speed, or flexibility.

• Weight-trained athletes use any form of progressive resistance exercise to improve their ability in a particular sport.

With this understanding, let's talk about the myths and misconceptions that have clouded the minds of non-weight-users concerning this activity.

1. Weight-lifters are ponderous and massive (maybe even fat), or grossly over-muscled. This misconception is the most galling of all to address, mainly because it would be so easy to correct if the TV and other media would realize what they have done and then correct this state of affairs.

There are nine classes in Olympic lifting (and as many in power-lifting), ranging from 114 pounds through 198, 242, and unlimited. But even during Olympic coverage, we rarely see any except the last two. Maybe it's because the bar bends more when the heavies lift (only a little more, though; the lighter classes are often within 50 pounds of the 500-plus jerk of the super-heavyweights), or maybe the media feel the sight of a 350-pound behemoth is more entertaining than that of a 114-pound flyweight efficiently handling close to three times his weight. Whatever the reason, they continue to promote the pre-1900 image of the strongman as slob.

The latest Olympic movie, *Visions of Eight,* perpetuates the same stereotype, even though the weight sequence is directed by woman filmmaker Mai Zetterling. Instead of slow side shots that could show a little of the grace and beauty of even the heaviest lifters, we are treated to close crops of contorted, fleshy faces and huge weights dropped in disgust. All this becomes nearly unbearable to anyone familiar with the sport, just as cliche photos of "agonizing" marathoners offend runners who love their sport.

The "gross" display of musculature we witness on Mr. Universe's appearing on the Johnny Carson show, for example, is way out of context. Such extreme muscularity takes years to attain, couldn't happen by accident, and may be observed only when such a display is intended (all the muscles flexed simultaneously). In suit and tie, or even in a tee-shirt, most body-builders look substantially more normal.

If any runner still fears such a fate might "accidentally" befall him, I give you this quote from John Jesse:

"Many track athletes have been led to believe that heavy resistance training automatically results in a large growth of muscle size. They fear that large muscles will hamper their speed and endurance development. Inherent body characteristics limit the amount of muscle or body size that can be developed.

"Ability to acquire large muscles is dependent to a great extend on the quantity of food intake, large amounts of sleep and rest, and a specific type of resistance exercise used by body-builders that builds large muscles and total body weight, with a relatively small increase in strength.

"The author (Jesse) has never seen a runner or hurdler who has worked with weights develop muscles of great size, as long as he participated in the type of endurance training required of him for success in his chosen event."

2. Weight-training makes you "muscle-bound." If by muscle-bound we mean inflexible, this is patently false and in most cases is the opposite of the effect we can expect. At the peak of my competitive lifting, I was also the most flexible I've ever been and was able to touch about 12 inches below my toes when standing on a bench.

Sam Loprinzi, who has lifted weights for more than 45 years and has been named Most Muscular Man and runner-up for Mr. America, can touch his head to the floor while sitting in a full split position. John C. Grimek, who lifted for the US Olympic team in 1936 and won Mr. America and Mr. Universe awards years later, could walk stiff-legged with his elbows touching the floor. At the peak of his career, with legs larger than the size of his contracted waist, Grimek could arch backwards into a handstand from a full split.

These are not rare exceptions but are typical of the total fitness these men strived for through weight training. With the elimination of the press from the Olympic lifts (and resulting elimination of the lower-back problems caused by the extreme backbend the press required), the modern lifter is getting slimmer and more flexible.

Yet a highly-paid *Sports Illustrated* writer recently misinformed his readers that a world record-holding Bulgarian lifter's elasticity is "unusual among lifters." Baloney! Such efforts are *due* to flexibility, and this flexibility is acquired through proper strength training, not despite it.

3. Weight-training hinders running speed or speed of reflexes. Both assumptions are false. An extreme example was Paul Anderson, the 375-pound Dixie Derrick who could run 100 yards in the 11's at this weight (some of which definitely was surplus). Numerous lighter lifters show much faster times, and strength training is now an accepted part of the program used by many sprinters to develop explosive starts and sustained drives.

In the area of reflexes, strength is seen to quicken them according to tests performed on different types of athletes by the US Army at the 1956 Olympics. Careful testing of the involved athletes clearly proved that a weight lifter had by far the fastest reflexes of those competing in any sport, and that most of the weight lifters were considerably faster than non lifters. With flexibility exercises, strength training does no harm to (and probably enhances) reflexes.

4. Weight-lifting is bad for women. This is an easy one. I could cite the long tradition of weight-training among women competing in the California beauty contest circuit or go into the physiological explanations involving differences of male and female hormones, but I'll simply cite a much more staid, mundane source—*Parade Magazine.* Reporting on experiments conducted by University of California exercise physiologist Jack Wilmore, *Parade* ran a feature article titled "Weight Lifting is for Women, too."

In a test covering 10 weeks, with each girl lifting weights in basic exercises for one hour three times a week, strength gains were reported for all subjects, ranging from 20-50%.

The size of waists, hips, and buttocks was reduced while bust size increased slightly—all positive results for women in American society. No change was reported in arm size or weight. The application to women runners is obvious. Unlike men, they don't even have to worry about gaining muscular bulk, while they can enjoy similar benefits from increases in strength.

5. Weight-lifters turn to flab when they quit working out. It didn't happen to me. My weight has been stable at 165 pounds over the last eight years. During a layoff my arms and legs decreased slightly in size, but my waist would increase by about an inch. This problem seems to be more a function of diet than exercise, and though muscle tissue can atrophy with lack of use and be replaced by fat, it is never a question of muscle turning to fat. Large muscles don't seem to lose very much tone if diet is adjusted to activity.

If I've established my point that strength training is not harmful to runners, I must go on to tell why it is a helpful—maybe even an essential—addition to their training.

To quote from *Sports Illustrated's Book of Track and Field: Running Events:* "We have said repeatedly that the best training for running is *running.* But there comes a time for every runner when an hour or so of weight lifting a week will do him more good and make him a better runner than another hour of running."

Here is the main reason why: *Balanced development can't be achieved by running alone.*

Running does very little to develop the upper body. Upper body power is obviously needed for the explosive sprint and hurdle events. And it can be very helpful at the end of longer races.

Dave Wottle, not overly muscled by any means at 6' 0", 140 pounds, is noted for his fine kick. Kenny Moore's *Sports Illustrated* article on Wottle makes the connection between his upper body strength and this strong kick: "His arms drop lower, and his surprising strength of torso (he can bench-press 180 pounds) churns him into another gear. 'The key is the arms,' he says. 'When I kick, all I do is concentrate on driving with my arms.'"

In the longer races like the marathon, upper body condition can pay off in the last miles of the race by reducing fatigue in the arms and shoulders, which can force the runner to slow his pace.

Running develops the legs, but in a very narrow way. The front of the leg gets proportionately stronger than the back of the leg, which increases chances for injury during unaccustomed stress. Another factor that can lead to injury is the fact that the leg is never fully straightened during running. (Motion studies show this, and the effect is more pronounced at a distance pace than in a sprint.) The result is a stiffness along the back of the leg, manifest in varying degrees from the buttock to the achilles tendon. Strength and flexibility training with emphasis on complete movements with full contractions can counter this tendency to stiffness while building power.

Finally, the vital midsection is best developed with vigorous calisthenics or progressive weight training.

Though anyone can profit from strength and flexibility training, it appears to become increasingly valuable with age, older people needing it more and seeing the preservation effects of such training more readily.

Now that I've had this partisan moment to defend the use of weights, I feel better about talking of the specific methods of weight training.

12

A Program for Runners
Charles Palmer

Rather than give examples of weight training programs that famous runners have used, it is more valuable for the individual runner to evaluate what parts of his body need work and to give enough exercises and variations so he can design his own program in a sensible manner. Weight lifters have long known that using a great number of exercises and variations produced better results than using a few motions repeatedly. Variety also tends to make training more enjoyable, of course.

The exercises that follow are listed according to the general body parts they affect, with variations noted where important. But, first, some general advice:

• **Equipment:** Except for two exercises, the only equipment needed is a barbell set (with adjustable dumbbells), a sit-up board, and stools or boxes (the board and boxes can be combined to make a bench needed for some movements). A 100-150 pound weight set is fine for a start. An iron set is preferable to the sand-filled plastic type, which is more bulky and wears out. Total cost will be comparable to that of a good pair of running shoes.

• **How often?** Two or three workouts a week is best, depending on how you react to the work load. Once a week is okay, but progress will be slower.

• **How much weight?** No one can say what you *should* do in each exercise. You'll determine this easily by experiment. For the first month, if you've never tried lifting weights before, you should stay very light and be more concerned with proper form than with how much you can lift. After this starting period, you should lift so you never have to strain to complete the number of repetitions you plan to do. Increase the weight when the poundage becomes easy, generally going up no more than five pounds at a time. Five percent every two weeks is a rough guideline to follow. Work hard but don't strain.

- **Breathing:** Breathe once per repetition, generally exhaling as the effort is performed but in the opposite phase if it feels better. Don't hold your breath longer than one repetition.

- **Number of exercises, sets, and repetitions:**

Exercises—Do from 5-10 per session, depending on how much time you can spend and how you react to the work. If you need more than the number you can do in a single session, split the schedule and repeat any exercises you feel are particularly important.

Sets—Aim for three per exercise with at least two sets per exercise, and up to four or five where you are weak.

Repetitions—This is an area where your own experiments are as important as the recommendations given with each movement. Low reps build power, high reps build endurance, but there is considerable overlap. Also, "high" and "low" are relative terms that may vary with the exercise.

You may choose to do all sets with the same number of repetitions or add weight to successive sets as you drop the reps (12-8-5 is a popular variation). Start each exercise with a set using a lower weight than you can normally handle for a given number of reps.

- **Sequence and rest pauses:** I favor running through each exercise completely before moving to the next, using one to two minutes rest between light exercises (for arms, shoulders, waist) and two to three minutes (or more as required) for heavy lifts involving large muscles (leg and back movements). However, I often run through the routine in cycles, moving from one exercise to the next with little rest between sets since the area being worked can recover during the work of the next exercise. This shortens the time spent per workout. Find what suits you best.

- **Boredom or stagnation at a certain weight:** Vary the exercise with a different hand-spacing, a reverse grip, or a different angle where this can be done. Vary the repetitions or sets if you find yourself going stale in a certain movement.

• **When to exercise:** Don't weight-train on days of very long runs or other hard running workouts. Upper body training can be done just before or after your regular running. Leg and back work should follow a running workout or precede it by several hours at least. Try to schedule a lifting workout no sooner than 1½ hours after a meal; finish no later than 30-45 minutes before big meals.

• **Dumbbells vs. barbells:** Some exercises favor the use of one over the other. Some have value when performed at different times using both types of weights. Barbells build basic strength. Dumbells force smaller supplementary muscles to work with larger, stronger muscles in coordinating the movement.

• **Warmup/substitute for weights:** Calisthenics are good for use in warming up for weight training, and there is a graduated program of these exercises that makes a fine five-minute warm-up or temporary conditioning exercises when you don't have access to weights. This is contained in the *Royal Canadian Air Force 5BX/XBX* program for men and women, available cheaply in paperback. Use this in the progressive manner described and you will be warmed up adequately for any weight training workouts, or you will retain fitness when you are unable to work out with weights.

One calisthenic exercise that requires no equipment yet can be done in a manner highly suited to the runner is the twisting sit-up. This is performed with feet flat on the floor, knees bent at about 90 degrees. The upper body curls up toward the thigh, starting from the head, and then the torso is twisted so the elbow falls outside the opposite knee, sides alternating with each repetition.

This sit-up approximates the twisting action the torso receives during running at any pace. For sprints, it can be done with weight behind the neck and on an inclined sit-up board (10-15 reps for power). For distance and conditoning, it can be done in sets of 20-100 reps with the feet held under a sofa or other heavy object.

One • Starting Position

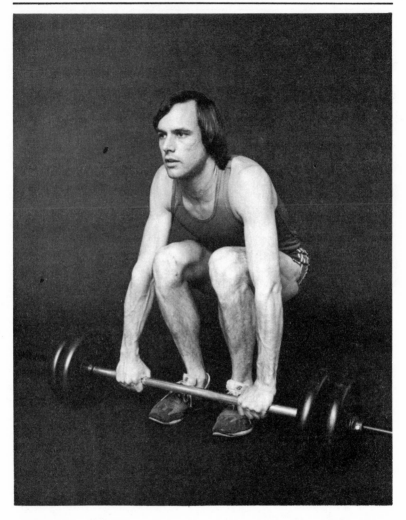

Basic Starting Position: Back straight, barbell close to ankles, hips low, arms straight, feet as flat as possible.

Two • Clean and Press

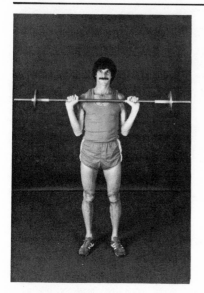 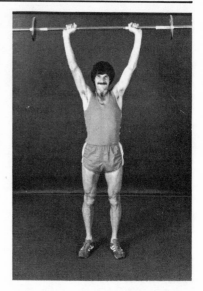

A. From **basic starting position,** straighten your legs until weight reaches knees. Snap the weight to shoulders using the back and continued leg straightening.

B. Push weight overhead with arms. Lower to shoulders. (Weight may also be lowered behind the head to shoulders, or dumbbells may be used. The "clean" alone may be performed as a back exercise and explosive power developer: 5-7 reps.)

Strengthens: Arms, shoulders, upper back.

Repetitions: 5-7 for power; 10 or more for endurance.

Three • Curl

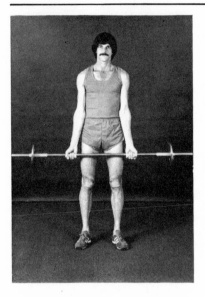 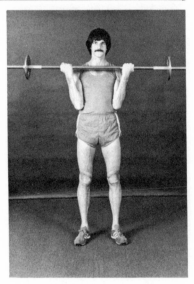

A. Weight hangs from arms, hands at shoulder-width with palms forward.

B. Curl weight to shoulders with the elbows stationary at sides. Be sure arms are completely straight as weight is lowered to repeat the lift. (Reverse curl is done with palms facing back, or dumbbells may be used.)

Strengthens: Biceps, forearms.

Repetitions: 5-7 reps for power; 10 or more for endurance.

Four • Upright Row

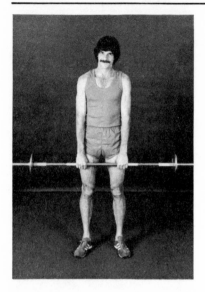 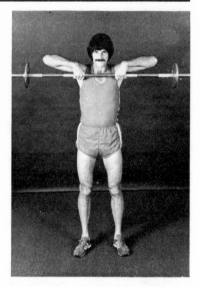

A. Hands about 8 inches apart, palms facing back, hands hanging in front.

B. Pull weight to shoulder level, using arms only—*no body swing.*

Strengthens: Biceps, shoulders, upper back.

Repetitions: 5-7 reps for power; 10-15 for endurance.

Five • Bent-Over Row

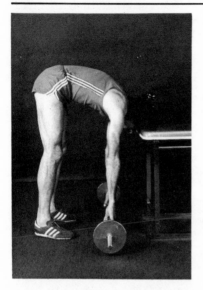 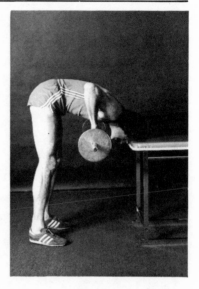

A. Legs slightly bent, body bent over with head braced on stool (optional) to eliminate body motion, back straight.

B. Pull bar up to touch middle of chest. (Variation: use single dumbbell with free hand braced on stool.)

Strengthens: Latissimus, trapezius, biceps and deltoids.

Repetitions: 7-10 reps for power; 12-20 reps for endurance.

Six • Bench Press

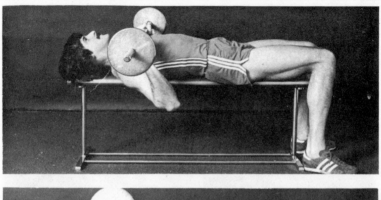

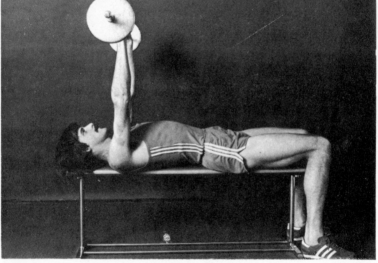

A. Lie flat on bench with barbell at the chest (you may need partner to assist with weight).

B. Press weight away from chest to complete extension.

Strengthens: Triceps, deltoids, pectorals.

Repetitions: 5-7 reps for power; 10-15 for endurance.

Seven • Bent-Arm Pullover

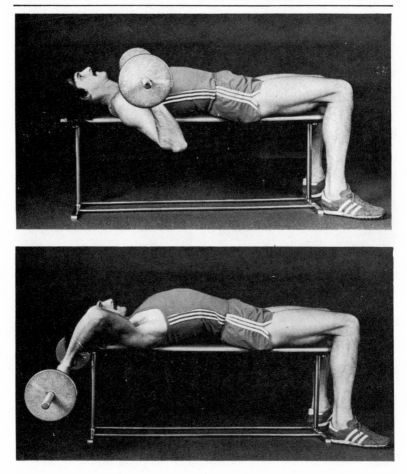

A. Start with narrow grip, weight resting high on chest.

B. Push weight back and down in an arc just over head. Allow weight to go below level of bench. Return to the chest. Perform in one smooth brisk cadence.

Strengthens: Pectorals, deltoids, arms.

Repetitions: 5-7 reps for power; 10-15 reps for endurance.

Eight • Arm-Swing

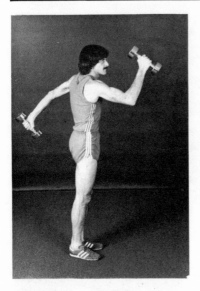 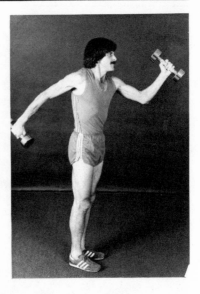

A. Hold light dumbbells in thumbs-up position. Alternate swinging of arms in rapid motion.

B. Back arm swings as far back as possible. Front arm bends to 90 degrees and comes up to eye level.

Strengthens: Arm, shoulder and upper back muscles used in running.

Repetitions: 7-10 cycles for power; 15-50 for endurance.

Nine • Stiff-Legged Dead Lift

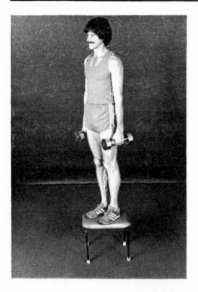 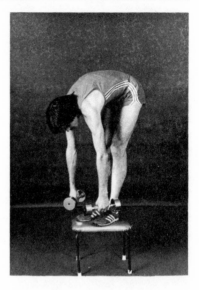

A. Start very slowly and carefully to avoid strain. Keep legs locked throughout.

B. Lower dumbbells (or barbell if flexibility doesn't permit touching toes with weight at first) to toes or below from elevated position on stool or box. Start with light weights and do not attempt to go very low at first. Proceed gradually.

Strengthens: Entire back and back of leg flexibility.

Repetitions: 10-20 reps for flexibility.

Ten • Side Bend

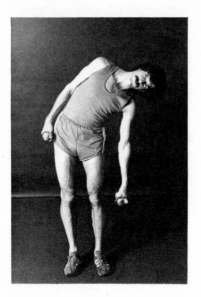 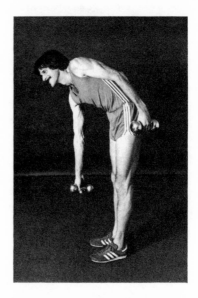

A. Hold dumbbells at sides and bend to each side alternately, as far as possible. Use very light weights to start. Work up to no more than 25-30 pounds. Increase reps after that point.

B. Variation: bend forward or arch backward during movement.

Strengthens: Lower back and sides.

Repetitions: At least 25 reps each direction.

Eleven • Toe Raise

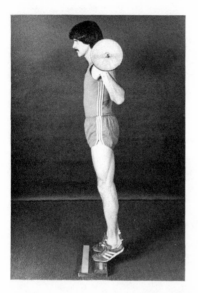 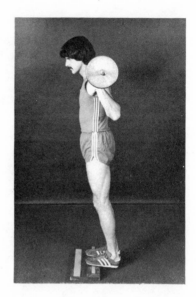

A. Use barbell—or single dumbbell if balance is hard to achieve. On elevated surface, rise up on toes as far as possible.

B. Then, lower as far as possible. Vary by turning feet in or out, or by balancing on one foot, then the other.

Strengthens: Calf muscles, Achilles tendon stretch.

Repetitions: 10-15 for power (with heavy weight) or flexibility (with low weight and complete stretch); 20-100 for endurance.

Twelve • Leg Kick

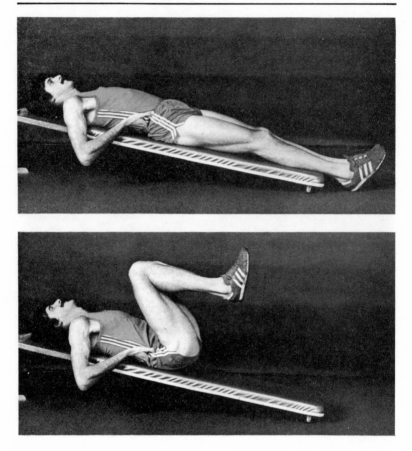

A. Lie flat on sit-up board (inclined for more resistance) with hands under hips.

B. Pull legs to chest.

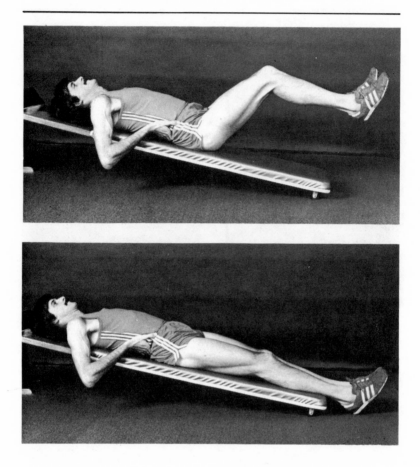

C. Extend legs . . .   **D.** Touching floor only at end of motion.

Strengthens: Lower abdominals and hip flexors.
Repetitions: 25-50 per set.

Thirteen • Bench Step

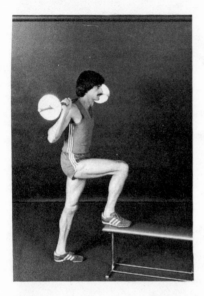 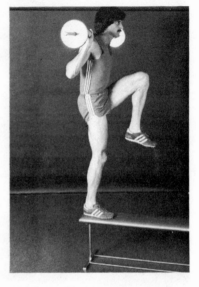

A. Step on bench or box 14-18 inches high, one leg straightening as the body is raised onto bench.

B. Draw up other leg to the chest as far as flexibility permits. Step down on same leg as you stepped up with.

Strengthens: Hips, thighs.

Repetitions: 7-10 reps for power; 15-25 for endurance.

Fourteen • Squat

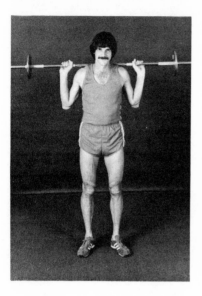 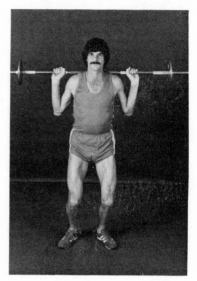

A. Begin with barbell in comfortable position on the shoulders, feet comfortably spaced and pointing outward.

B. Drop to partial squat, or . . .

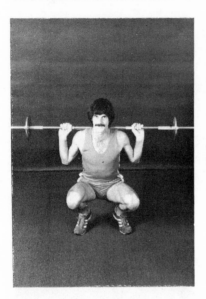 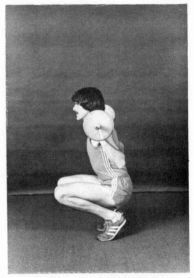

C. To a full squat. (Don't bounce into full squat.) Use board under heels if Achilles flexibility does not permit keeping heels flat throughout movement.

D. Side view of full squat position.

Strengthens: Hips, thighs, hamstrings.

Repetitions: 5-10 reps of partial squat for power; 15-25 for endurance. Never do less than 15 of full squat; preferably 20-25 for endurance.

Fifteen • Leg Curl

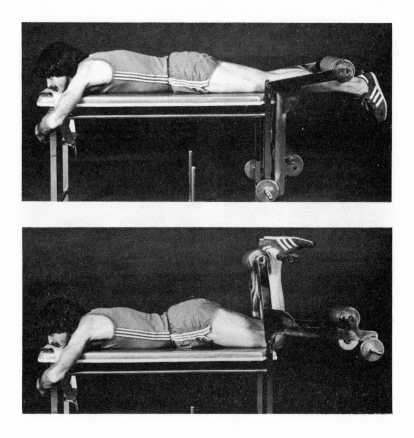

A. Lie flat on stomach on leg curl/extension machine or with "iron boots" that strap to shoes.

B. Swinging legs forward smoothly, be certain there is full contraction and extension with each movement.

Strengthens: Hamstrings.

Repetitions: 7-12 reps for power; 15-30 for endurance.

Sixteen • Leg Extensions

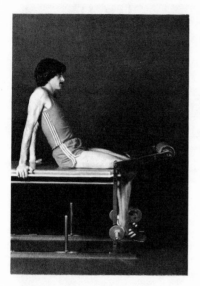 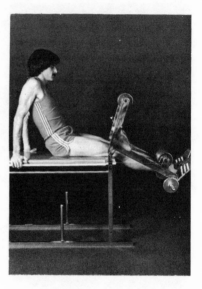

A. Performed on the same equipment as leg curls.

B. Do repetitions smoothly with swinging motions. Be sure there is full contraction and full extension with each movement.

Strengthens: Quadriceps.

Repetitions: 7-12 reps for power; 15-30 for endurance.

13

Fifty-Minute Supplement
Wayne Roe

Like milk, running is often considered the "complete physical food," packing stamina, strength, muscle tone, cardiovascular development, mental relaxation. and a myriad of other "nutrients" in a single, inexpensive activity.

I'm not disputing this idea. Indeed, I fully agree with it. I only wish to prescribe a simple supplement to a regular running diet that will promote optimal physical development and reduce the incidence of running-related injuries.

Recently, I began to suffer the symptoms of overdevelopment of the legs, a common ailment of runners. Three years of long slow distance, interval training and frequent racing had made my legs tight and produced a succession of injuries to my calves and achilles tendons. Additionally, I frequently experienced a lack of general physical strength in workouts and paces, which detracted from my enjoyment and inhibited my performance. I resolved to correct this defect in my training program with minimal extra time and effort. Having become familiar with stretching exercises and weight training in my youth and through two years of karate, I assembed a program requiring but 50 minutes a week. It has more than fulfilled its promise.

I realize that many runners are skeptical of the value of exercises such as weight training and stretching. Such skepticism in part underlies the failure of many to warm up and warm down properly, a major contributor to injuries and poor performances. Perhaps even more importantly, it indicates a lack of knowledge of the potential and limitations of one's body, which I feel is an important dividend of any

---

Wayne Roe has written about weight training for runners in *Runner's World*. A marathoner, he ran the 1976 Boston Marathon in 2:31 and the 1977 New York City Marathon in 2:28.

physical activity. My 50 minutes a week has left me free from injuries and has given me a wealth of self-knowledge.

A law of weight training states: heavy weights, few repetitions build strength; light weights and many repetitions build stamina. My program incorporates the best of both approaches. It produces strength and endurance without the bulky muscles, that can inhibit the fluidity of one's stride.

I began my program while I was a student at Michigan State University and had access to a Universal weight machine. Consequently the exercises are tailored to some extent to this equipment. Most colleges and many high schools have such a machine, its advantage being speed in changing the weight settings. Any set of barbells will work just as well, however, and barbells are convenient and private.

The workout I prescribe is extremely short, simple, and so structured that each exercise becomes progressively easier to complete. It begins with a five-minute stretching session.

After one minute of rest, the weight session begins. The exercises are specifically for the upper body. I feel that my legs get enough of a workout in daily running training, but some runners may need additional leg exercises. Four separate exercises comprise the weight workout: (1) the military (overhead) press, (2) the two-armed curl, (3) the bench press, and (4) the overhead pull (or rowing exercise if one uses conventional barbells). Anyone not familiar with the form of these exercises will find descriptions earlier in this chapter and in other weight training books.

At the beginning, you must find a personal "maximizing weight" for each exercise and set an upper limit on the loads which one works with. The maximizing weight is the heaviest weight one can lift in a given exercise for eight repetitions. Take care not to incur undue strain in determining this figure. There should be an effort to lift, but not a tooth-and-nail struggle. Subtract 20 pounds from each of your four maximums, and you arrive at the starting points of each exercise.

As an example, my personal starting points are 100 pounds for the military press, 70 pounds for the curl, 130 pounds for the bench press, and 110 pounds for the overhead pull. Remember: It is better to be lifting too light rather than too heavy at the start. Everyone will progress, but weights—like running—take time to shower benefits.

The program is designed to produce maximal strength and muscular endurance to the distance runner. One will not experience a bulking of the upper body, but at most a slight increase in muscular definition, which does not inhibit the fluidity of one's stride.

Each exercise is performed only once during the course of a workout for a total of 40 repetitions. Beginning with the starting weight, do 10 repetitions of one exercise and then immediately (no rest) reduce the load 20 pounds and do 10 reps, then another 20-pound reduction and 10 reps, and still one more set with 20 pounds less. Then take a two-minute rest before proceeding to the next exercise.

The format, 10 reps times four sets, is the same for each exercise; only the starting points differ. The recommended order of the exercises is (1) military press, (2) curl, (3) bench press, (4) pull. Do each set as rapidly as possible. This helps build muscular endurance, a valuable asset at the end of a race or workout when arm motion "carries" you. Make sure to pace yourself so that all repetitions can be completed at each weight level, however.

Properly done, the stretching-weight workout I have outlined requires no more than 20-25 minutes to complete. I do it three times a week, although two sessions are adequate for most runners. A fundamental rule of weight training is to take at least one day of rest between workouts. Monday-Thursday or some other two-day rest schedule seems best.

What results should you expect from the program which I have outlined?

First, one must remember that weight training takes time to produce significant results, two to three months minimum. Consequently, you must follow it as religiously as your running regimen to get the full benefits. A missed workout here and there will not hurt, but too many days off will result in a loss of physical and mental stamina.

I have easily incorporated this program in my daily workouts without any adverse effects. I might add that I feel best when the weight work is done before running. For a few minutes I experience a tight, fatigued feeling as I begin running but this abates in a mile or so. I have run many of my best interval and distance workouts after lifting weights.

After three months, the runner following my program should have experienced a number of physical and psychological benefits. His strength will be far greater and much more "balanced" than before. It has been said that "speed is strength," and there should be definite gains in this department. Perhaps because of my ability to maintain faster and more relaxed armswings, my short distance times have significantly improved from weight work. The addition of upper body strength helps "carry" me through workouts and races when the legs start to break down. Purely the addition of this workout to my training diet brought my marathon time down from 3:15 to 2:55, and made the "last six" much easier to run.

The combination of weights and stretching has also produced a remarkable freedom from injury in my own case. Since beginning this program, my log shows no days off due to injury, while before this time I could count on four days off per month as a minimum.

Finally, there are untold psychological benefits which should come from this program. Weight training reduces flab and promotes muscle tone and definition. One looks and feels better and naturally is more confident. It is almost impossible not to run better under these conditions.

I realize that most runners feel that a pure running diet is sufficient for the conditioning needs of their bodies. Most would prefer to spend the 50 minutes my program takes on the road or the track. I believe, however, that the additional 6-8 miles per week one would gain are far outweighted by the benefits of my program, especially in the defense against injury which it promotes. Personal experience bears me out on this point.

I encourage all of my running compatriots to experiment with this program for three months or so, perhaps beginning in the winter when the extra miles will not be missed as much. Even the "complete food" will have been supplemented.

V
Weight Training for Women

14
Weights for Women
Bob Hyten

The Ozark Track Club of greater St. Louis is one of the
few women's teams which has weight lifting in its regular
training schedule. While I make no claims that this is an
ultimate program or even that it is 100% correct, it is the
result of three years of refinement and has given us positive results.

The purpose of the program is to develop all-around
strength and endurance. There is no attempt to build muscle
bulk. The emphasis is on the kind of strength that results
in quickness and spring while carrying the body in a relaxed
manner. It is designed to eliminate tired arms in distance
runners and weak backs in high jumpers, plus developing
strong ankles and calves for long jumpers and overall leg
strength for hurdlers—all the while keeping the figures in
mind. One basis for settling on the program is that it is of
value to all members of the team. I should note that all
members learn every event, and most of them regularly com-
pete in the pentathlon.

I limit weight lifting to those women whose growth has
leveled off. Muscles being stretched by rapid growth do not
need the further strain of being tightened by lifting. I do let
the younger women do some of the arm work during our
group practices because almost all women are too weak to
carry their arms through a race.

The majority of our lifting is confined to our development
seasons—August through March or cross-country and indoor
seasons. Good cross-country runners do little or no lifting
in the main part of their season, but since we attach little

Bob Hyten has coached with the Ozark Track Club, one of the
strongest Midwestern girls' and womens' teams, and the United States
Association. He also coached Judy Vernon, 1972 British Olympian,
and 1974 Commonwealth hurdles champion.

importance to the short indoor season all do their major lifting at that time. Lifting is done three days a week (every other day) from Dec. 1 to April 1, then is gradually phased out during April. Full-scale running workouts aimed at development of strength and endurance are done on the alternate days.

Intense running, warm-up and stretching sessions precede weight lifting. We do 12 different lifts or exercises in about the same order each time. The variance from the order comes when we do sets of arm exercises between sets of leg exercises in order to fully utilize our equipment as well as keep the sessions from dragging out too long.

One • Half-Squats

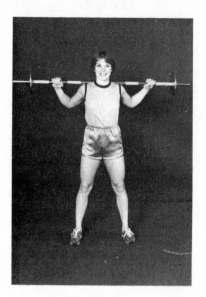 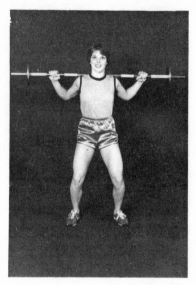

A. Barbell rests at shoulder, legs spread comfortably as starting position.

B. Squat halfway to knees, keeping barbell level.

Strengthens: Thighs.

Suggested Weight: 40 lbs. Add 10 every 4th session up to a limit of 1½ times body weight.

Repetitions: 3 sets of 10.

Two • 3-in-1 • Two-Arm Curl

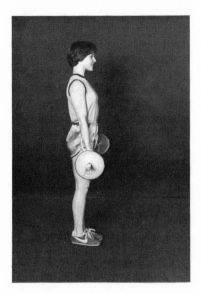

A. Use shoulder-width undergrip with barbell across upper-thighs. Make sure feet are spread comfortably for good balance.

B. Holding elbows in tight to torso, curl bar up to chin.

Strengthens: Biceps, shoulders, triceps.

Suggested Weight: 10 lbs. Increase by every 4th session to a maximum of 40-50 lbs.

Repetitions: 1 set of 10, each done consecutively.

3-in-1 • Upright Rowing Exercise

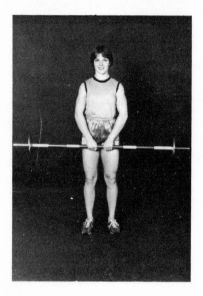 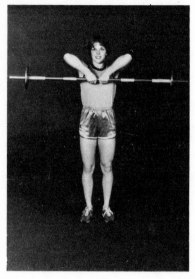

A. Narrow grip, palms in, weight at thighs.

B. Lift barbell to chin, keeping the elbows high, and trying as best you can to keep bar level.

Strengthens: Biceps, shoulders, triceps.

Suggested Weight: 10 lbs. Increase by every 4th session to a maximum of 40-50 lbs.

Repetitions: 1 set of 10, each done consecutively.

3-in-1 • Two-Hand Press Exercise

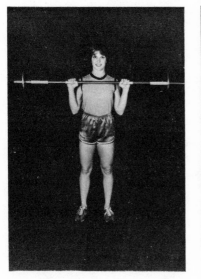 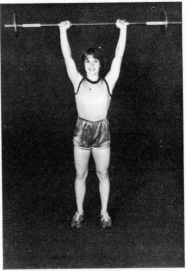

A. Start with the barbell at shoulder height, hands shoulder-width apart.

B. Lift barbell to full overhead extension. Return to shoulder level and repeat.

Strengthens: Biceps, shoulders, triceps.

Suggested Weight: 10 lbs. Increase by every 4th session to a maximum of 40-50 lbs.

Repetitions: 1 set of 10, each done consecutively.

Three • Leg Extensions

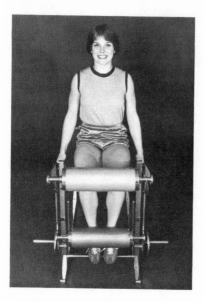

A. Sitting on the end of the leg-extension table, hook instep under bottom roller. Feet aimed straight forward.

B. Under weight resistance, straighten legs and hold for a few seconds (15 seconds on last of each set).

Strengthens: Frontal thighs.

Suggested Weight: 20 lbs. Raise by 5 every 7th session.

Repetitions: 3 sets of 10.

Four • Wrist Curls

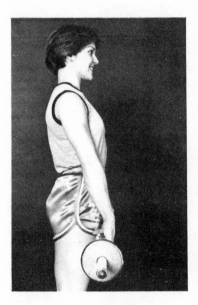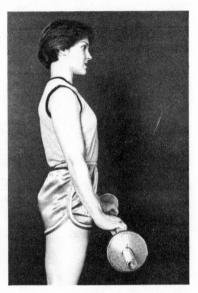

A. Using a shoulder-width overgrip, roll the bar inward using wrist strength only.

B. Flexing again at wrists only, curl bar upward as high as possible.

Strengthens: Wrists, forearms.

Suggested Weight: 10 lbs.

Repetitions: 5 reps, no increase.

Five • Sit-Ups

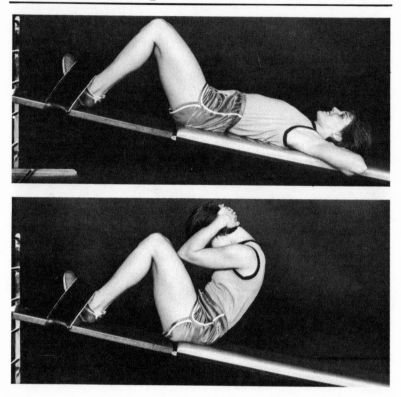

A. Do the bent-leg sit-ups on a slight incline.

B. Curl body upward until elbows meet knees. These kinds of sit-ups will flatten the stomach and strengthen the diaphragm for breathing. (*Hint:* Always keep the legs bent and slightly unlocked to keep strain off lower back.)

Strengthens: Abdominal muscles.

Suggested Weight: None to start. After 30 can be accomplished easily, add 2½ lbs. behind head, then 5, finally 10.

Repetitions: One set of 30.

Six • Back Curls

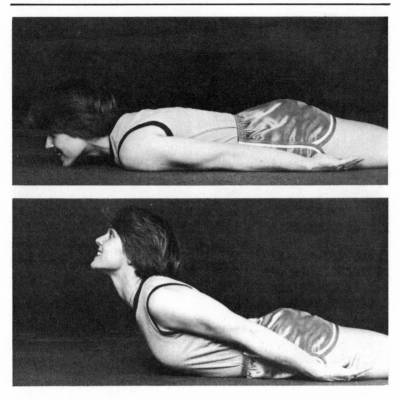

A. Lie on stomach, feet supported by a partner or a bench apparatus.

B. Raise upper body.

Strengthens: Lumbar musculature.

Repetitions: One set of 30.

Seven • Split Squats

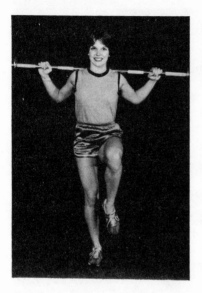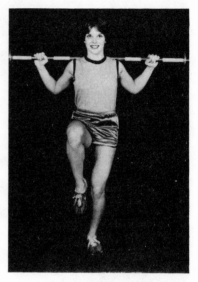

A. With weight on shoulder, jump into air off left foot, balancing on right.

B. Then jump off the right foot, balancing on left.

Strengthens: Thighs, calves.

Suggested Weight: One-half of half-squat weight (20 lbs.).

Repetitions: One set of 20 jumps (10 on each foot).

Eight • Bench Press

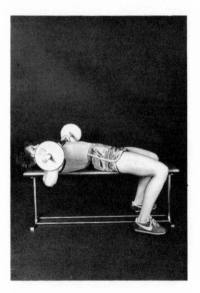 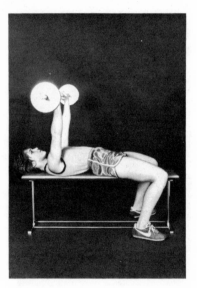

A. Lie flat, feet planted on floor and overgrip on bar.

B. Raise (press) to arm's length.

Strengthens: Chest (pectorals).

Suggested Weight: 20 lbs., increasing 5 each 4th session, to a maximum for runners of about 40-50 lbs.

Repetitions: 3 sets of 10.

Nine • Toe (Heel) Raises

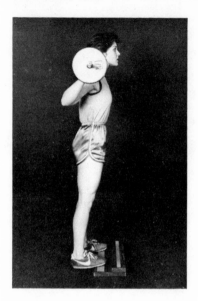 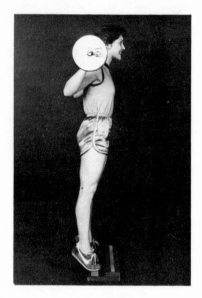

A. Stand on a two-by-four board with ball of foot and toes, the weight balanced on shoulders.

B. Raise up on the toes as high as possible. Do first set with heels parallel; second with toes together and heels out; and third with heels together and toes out.

Strengthens: Calf muscles.

Suggested Weight: 40 lbs.

Repetitions: 3 sets of 10.

Ten • Groin

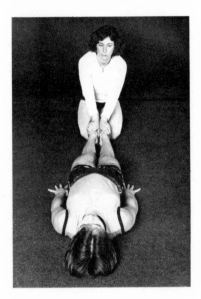 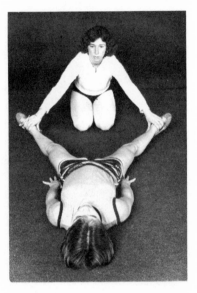

A. Lie on back, with legs straight, feet together. Your partner should hold your ankles firmly.

B. Try to spread legs while your partner offers resistance. Then (partner still resisting) return legs to the starting position.

Strengthens: Leg, groin muscles.

Repetitions: 1 set of 10.

Eleven • Hamstring

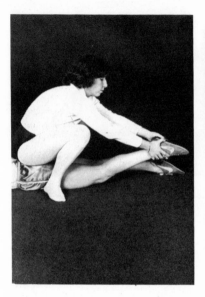 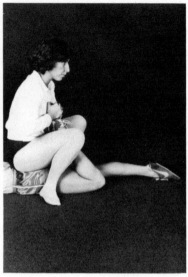

A. Lie face down, partner seated as shown.

B. As partner offers resistance against the ankle, raise leg toward buttocks. Lower leg the same way.

Strengthens: Hamstrings.

Repetitions: 1 set of 10 (each leg).

Twelve • Good Morning Exercise

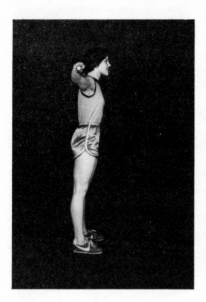 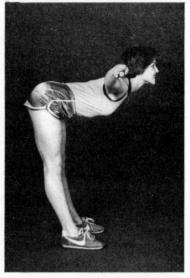

A. Start with the bar across your shoulders and feet a comfortable distance apart.

B. From this erect position and with legs locked out, bend over 90 degrees, and recover to starting position.

Strengthens: Lower back, hamstrings.

Suggested Weight: Bar alone to 10 lbs.

Repetitions: 1 set of 10.

Thirteen • Leg Curl

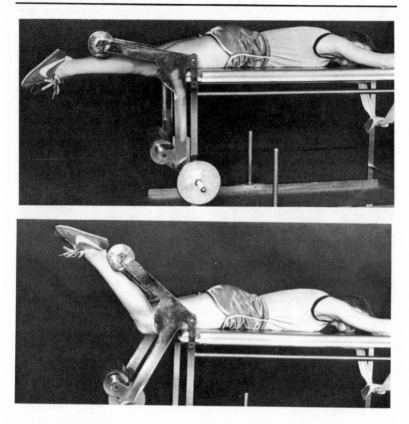

A. Lie face down on the leg extension table, heels curled under the roller.

B. Bend the legs as much as possible. Then return them to the starting position. To get the widest arc possible, it might be necessary to hold on to the table to keep upper body position.

Strengthens: Hamstrings.

Suggested Weight: 20 lbs. to start.

Repetitions: 3 sets of 10.

Acknowledgments

Bob Wischnia, Assistant editor of *Runner's World* and Senior editor of *Marathoner* magazine, posed for the Six Flexibility Tests.

Jill Benyo began running in her mid-20s when she moved to California. She runs 10-15 miles per week during a busy schedule of working, acting, and ballet classes and occasional low-key weekend races.

Jean McWilliams Couch, who posed for the yoga asanas and wrote the captions, has been studying yoga for six years and is presently a student at the Institute of Yoga Teacher Education in San Francisco. She teaches yoga at the Palo Alto YMCA and for various industries and private groups.

Duncan MacDonald includes weight training as an integral part of his overall training schedule. One of America's most versatile distance runners, he is a former US 5000 meter record-holder, a 2:17 marathoner (West Valley), and winner of the 1976 Honolulu Marathon.

Edie Leen, our woman weight trainer, is a gym instructor, model, and current holder of the title "Miss Bay Area Body Beautiful." She runs 25 miles each week to complement her weight training program.

Photographs by **Dave Madison.**

Thanks to the **Lydia Young Health Spa,** Los Altos, California, for the use of their weight training facilities.

Index